Current and New Techniques for Primary and Revision Arthrodesis

Guest Editor

BEAT HINTERMANN, MD

FOOT AND ANKLE CLINICS

www.foot.theclinics.com

Consulting Editor
MARK S. MYERSON, MD

March 2011 • Volume 16 • Number 1

SAUNDERS an imprint of ELSEVIER, Inc.

W.B. SAUNDERS COMPANY
A Division of Elsevier Inc.

1600 John F. Kennedy Blvd. ● Suite 1800 ● Philadelphia, PA 19103-2899

http://www.theclinics.com

FOOT AND ANKLE CLINICS Volume 16, Number 1
March 2011 ISSN 1083-7515, ISBN-13: 978-1-4557-0447-7

Editor: Debora Dellapena
Developmental Editor: Jessica Demetriou

Foot and Ankle Clinics (ISSN 1083-7515) is published quarterly by Elsevier, Inc., 360 Park Avenue South, New York, NY 10010-1710. Months of issue are March, June, September, and December. Periodicals postage paid at New York, NY, and additional mailing offices. Subscription price per year is $271.00 (US individuals), $357.00 (US institutions), $134.00 (US students), $308.00 (Canadian individuals), $422.00 (Canadian institutions), $184.00 (Canadian students), $397.00 (foreign individuals), $422.00 (foreign institutions), and $184.00 (foreign students). To receive student/resident rate, orders must be accompanied by name of affiliated institution, date of term, and the *signature* of program/residency coordinator on institution letterhead. Orders will be billed at individual rate until proof of status is received. Foreign air speed delivery is included in all *Clinics* subscription prices. All prices are subject to change without notice. **POSTMASTER:** Send address changes to *Foot and Ankle Clinics*, Elsevier Health Sciences Division, Subscription Customer Service, 3251 Riverport Lane, Maryland Heights, MO 63043. **Customer Service: 1-800-654-2452 (US and Canada). From outside of the United States and Canada, call 314-447-8871. Fax: 314-447-8029. E-mail: JournalsCustomerService-usa@ elsevier.com (for print support); JournalsOnlineSupport-usa@elsevier.com (for online support).**

Reprints. For copies of 100 or more, of articles in this publication, please contact the Commercial Reprints Department, Elsevier Inc., 360 Park Avenue South, New York, NY 10010-1710. Tel.: 212-633-3812; Fax: 212-462-1935; E-mail: reprints@elsevier.com.

Printed and bound by CPI Group (UK) Ltd, Croydon, CR0 4YY

Transferred to Digital Print 2011

Contributors

CONSULTING EDITOR

MARK S. MYERSON, MD
Director, Institute for Foot and Ankle Reconstruction at Mercy, Mercy Medical Center, Baltimore, Maryland

GUEST EDITOR

BEAT HINTERMANN, MD
Chairman, Associate Professor, Clinic of Orthopaedic and Trauma Surgery, Kantonsspital Liestal, Switzerland

AUTHORS

FRANK R. AVILUCEA, MD
Resident, Department of Orthopaedics, University of Utah, Salt Lake City, Utah

ALEXEJ BARG, MD
Resident, Clinic of Orthopaedic Surgery, Kantonsspital Liestal, Liestal, Switzerland; Research Fellow, Harold K. Dunn Orthopaedic Research Laboratory, University Orthopaedic Center, Salt Lake City, Utah

TIMOTHY BEALS, MD
Associate Professor, Department of Orthopaedics, University of Utah, Salt Lake City, Utah

SAMUEL BRUNNER, MD
Attending Surgeon, Clinic of Orthopaedic Surgery, Kantonsspital Liestal, Liestal, Switzerland

MICHAEL P. CLARE, MD
Director of Fellowship Education, Foot and Ankle Fellowship, Florida Orthopaedic Institute, Tampa, Florida

BRIAN E. CLOWERS, MD
Fellow, The Institute for Foot and Ankle Reconstruction, Mercy Medical Center, Baltimore, Maryland

JANET D. CONWAY, MD
Rubin Institute for Advanced Orthopedics, International Center for Limb Lengthening, Sinai Hospital of Baltimore, Baltimore, Maryland

XAVIER CREVOISIER, MD, PD
President of the Swiss Foot and Ankle Society, Médecin Chef Site Hôpital Orthopédique, Department of Orthopedic Surgery, Centre Hospitalier Universitaire Vaudois, Lausanne, Switzerland

NORMAN ESPINOSA, MD
Head of Foot and Ankle Surgery, Department of Orthopaedics, University of Zurich, Balgrist, Zurich, Switzerland

PATRICIO FUENTES CARVAJAL, MD
Clínica Santa María, Providencia, Santiago, Chile

RENÉE A. FUHRMANN, MD
Department of Foot and Ankle Surgery, Rhön-Klinikum, Bad Neustadt, Germany

BEAT HINTERMANN, MD
Chairman, Associate Professor, Clinic of Orthopaedic and Trauma Surgery, Kantonsspital Liestal, Switzerland

MARKUS KNUPP, MD
Department of Orthopaedic Surgery, Kantonsspital Liestal, Liestal, Switzerland

STEPHEN J. LIPSCOMBE, MRCS
Specialist Registrar in Orthopaedics, Department of Orthopaedics and Trauma, University Hospital Aintree, Liverpool, United Kingdom

ANDY P. MOLLOY, FRCS (Tr&Orth)
Consultant Orthopaedic Surgeon, Department of Orthopaedics and Trauma, University Hospital Aintree, Liverpool, United Kingdom

GERARDO MUÑOZ MURARO, MD, PhD
Departamento de Traumatología, Clínica Las Condes, Las Condes, Santiago, Chile

MARK S. MYERSON, MD
Director, Institute for Foot and Ankle Reconstruction at Mercy, Mercy Medical Center, Baltimore, Maryland

FLORIAN NICKISCH, MD
Assistant Professor, Department of Orthopaedics, University of Utah, Salt Lake City, Utah

CHARLES SALTZMAN, MD
Professor and Chair, Department of Orthopaedics, University of Utah, Salt Lake City, Utah

ROY W. SANDERS, MD
Director, Orthopaedic Trauma Service, Tampa General Hospital, Florida Orthopaedic Institute, Tampa, Florida

REINHARD SCHUH, MD
Foot and Ankle Center Vienna, Vienna; Department of Orthopaedic Surgery, Innsbruck Medical University, Innsbruck, Austria

KALPESH S. SHAH, MS, FRCS Tr Orth
Clinical Fellow, Foot and Ankle Surgery, St Paul's Hospital, Vancouver, British Columbia, Canada

SJOERD A.S. STUFKENS, MD
Department of Orthopaedic Surgery, Academic Medical Center, Amsterdam, The Netherlands

RISHI THAKRAL, MBBS, ARFCS, MCh, MSc(Orth Eng), FRCSI (Tr&Orth)
Rubin Institute for Advanced Orthopedics, International Center for Limb Lengthening, Sinai Hospital of Baltimore, Baltimore, Maryland

HANS-JOERG TRNKA, MD
Associate Professor, Foot and Ankle Center Vienna, Vienna, Austria

STEPHAN H. WIRTH, MD
Consultant, Foot and Ankle Surgery, Department of Orthopaedics, University of Zurich, Balgrist, Zurich, Switzerland

ALASTAIR S. YOUNGER, ChM, MD
Director, Foot and Ankle Clinic, Department of Foot and Ankle Surgery, University of British Columbia; Associate Professor, Department of Foot and Ankle Surgery, St Paul's Hospital, Vancouver, British Columbia, Canada

ALAN J. ZONNO, MD
Fellow, The Institute for Foot and Ankle Reconstruction, Mercy Medical Center, Baltimore, Maryland

LUKAS ZWICKY, MSc
Research Fellow, Clinic of Orthopaedic Surgery, Kantonsspital Liestal, Liestal, Switzerland

Contents

Based on a high percentage of good results, retrospective studies strongly suggest that isolated talonavicular arthrodesis provides efficient pain relief and functional improvement in case of talonavicular arthritis in rheumatoid arthritis, primary or posttraumatic arthritis, flexible acquired flatfoot deformity, residual dorsolateral subluxation of the talonavicular joint after surgical treatment of clubfoot, and some neurologic disorders. However, prospective trials with rigorous methodology are required to establish evidence of efficacy for this procedure. Well-designed biomechanical studies have demonstrated the key role of the talonavicular joint in the complex hindfoot motion and may serve as baseline for further prospective studies.

Triple arthrodesis is largely used to restore painful hindfoot deformity. However, the procedure has been connected to several postoperative complications. Therefore, an isolated fusion of the talonavicular and the subtalar joint through a single medial approach has gained popularity. This "diple" arthrodesis provides effective correction of deformities and reduces the risk of wound healing problems on the lateral side of the foot.

Combined subtalar and naviculocuneiform fusion was successful in restoring the longitudinal medial arch after extended breakdown while preserving the talon avicular joint. This surgical technique was shown to give a reliable fusion and biomechanically stable position of the foot. In this review article, we summarize the medial column procedures for flatfoot deformity and present our surgical technique and results of 10 consecutive patients treated with this method at a minimum 1-year follow-up.

Isolated subtalar arthrodesis is well accepted for treatment of pathologic conditions of the subtalar joint associated with pain, instability, and deformity that do not respond to conservative treatment. The most frequent indications are primary talocalcaneal or posttraumatic arthrosis; congenital malformations (coalition); or inflammatory diseases. In the last years, arthroscopic subtalar arthrodesis has become an established technique in treatment of the subtalar arthrosis in the absence of deformities, misalignment and bone loss. As this technique limits soft tissue damages, it may diminish hospitalization days. However, this technique necessitates basic experience in arthroscopy of small joints and knowledge of specific anatomy.

examination and imaging are crucial for accurate preoperative planning. If performed, successful outcomes can be achieved with the strategies outlined in this article.

The use of a spherical femoral head allograft in conjunction with spherical reaming provides a safe and effective technique for the management of a massive osseous defect in the hindfoot. This technique presents specific advantages over the standard technique of trapezoidal block allograft and joint preparation by way of flat osteotomies, including increased flexibility and freedom in deformity correction and joint alignment.

THE CLINICS ARE NOW AVAILABLE ONLINE!

Access your subscription at:
www.theclinics.com

Preface

Current and New Techniques for Primary and Revision Arthrodesis

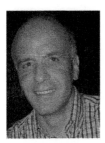

Beat Hintermann, MD
Guest Editor

Arthrodesis of the foot and ankle has been used to treat a variety of neuromuscular and degenerative foot disorders for more than 100 years. Techniques have evolved over time, and well-designed biomechanical studies have provided guidance regarding the desirable ranges of foot alignment during arthrodesis. As contemporary implants have made osseous union more reliable, indications and techniques for the fusion of selected joints have evolved and offer the promise of improved function. Nonetheless, the underlying principles of careful tissue handling, meticulous joint alignment, and attentive aftercare remain important in these complex procedures. The method of fixation must be considered, as this may determine the type of arthrodesis that is required.

The complex nature of these conditions makes it difficult for a single surgeon to become adept in dealing with the multitude of pathologies and available techniques. The authors in this issue of *Foot and Ankle Clinics of North America* are experts in dealing with complex pathologies requiring a stable and well-aligned foot and ankle, each one specializing in a unique condition and fixation technique. They all provide experienced insight into the appropriate management of these challenging problems, whether common or uncommon. By sharing the knowledge and experience of our colleagues, each of us can expand our ability to treat these complex conditions.

I would like to commend the international authors on the tremendous time and effort that they put forth in preparation of their articles. I would like to thank Dr Myerson and everyone at Elsevier for their help in putting this issue together. We hope that our

Foot Ankle Clin N Am 16 (2011) xiii–xiv
doi:10.1016/j.fcl.2011.01.005
1083-7515/11/$ – see front matter © 2011 Elsevier Inc. All rights reserved.

foot.theclinics.com

efforts will assist in the treatment of patients, leading ultimately to improved results and quality of life.

Beat Hintermann, MD
Clinic of Orthopaedic and Trauma Surgery
Kantonsspital Liestal
Rheinstrasse 26
CH-4410, Switzerland

E-mail address:
beat.hintermann@ksli.ch

First Metatarsophalangeal Arthrodesis for Hallux Rigidus

Renée A. Fuhrmann, MD

KEYWORDS

• Hallux rigidus • Arthrodesis • Metatarsophalangeal joint

Hallux rigidus leads to a restricted and painful motion at the first metatarsophalangeal (MTP 1) joint. The symptoms mainly occur in the final phase of the gait cycle (push-off phase), when the toes are passively forced in dorsiflexion. The underlying pathologic condition is discussed controversially. Altered biomechanics of the MTP 1 joint (lack of gliding motion during dorsiflexion) may be attributed both to the dorsal osteophytes at the metatarsal head and to a contracture of the plantar soft tissues involving the sesamoids. Therefore, pain is prompted by standing on tiptoes, climbing stairs, and wearing shoes with high heels or a flexible sole. Additional discomfort results from dorsal osteophytes at the metatarsal head, which lead to shoe-fitting problems involving local pressure, bursitis, and skin irritation.

To avoid painful joint motion at the MTP 1 joint, patients try to reduce load bearing at the first ray by active supination of the foot. Consequently, the hallux disorder leads to lateralization of load bearing during propulsion, which may result in transfer metatarsalgia and painful plantar callosities.

If conservative measures (such as use of rocker bottom shoes, intra-articular corticoid injections) fail, operative procedures can be taken into consideration. Decision making of the appropriate surgical procedure mainly refers to the stage of hallux rigidus. Advanced stages of osteoarthritis can be addressed by resection arthroplasty, joint replacement, or arthrodesis. The differential indication is influenced by the patient's age and physical demands, the underlying cause, concomitant diseases, and the surgeon's personal experience.

Arthrodesis of the MTP 1 joint (first described by Clutton in 1894) is widely accepted as the gold standard for end-stage hallux rigidus. Furthermore, patients with painful and stiff MTP 1 joints benefit from arthrodesis, even if the radiological arthritic changes are minor. Fusion results in a reliable clinical outcome with obvious biomechanical

The author has not received any funding support and has nothing to disclose.
Department of Foot and Ankle Surgery, Rhön-Klinikum, Salzburger Leite 1, 97616 Bad Neustadt, Germany
E-mail address: RAEFuhrmann@aol.com

foot.theclinics.com

benefits. With the MTP 1 joint arthrodesis performed in an appropriate position (25° dorsiflexion), the medial ray is stabilized, so that even the windlass mechanism works.[1]

However, fusion of the MTP 1 joint limits the use of fashionable footwear and alters the gait. Gait analysis after MTP 1 joint arthrodesis revealed a significant decrease in step length, plantar flexion of the ankle, and power at the push-off phase.[2,3]

PREOPERATIVE CONSIDERATIONS

The physical examination should not be limited to the MTP 1 joint. It is essential to further evaluate the entire foot (hindfoot alignment), neurovascular status, first interphalangeal (IP 1) joint, and adjacent lesser toes.

Standard radiographs include weight-bearing anteroposterior and lateral views; oblique views are optional. If women insist on wearing special shoes, a lateral radiograph may be taken in the standard shoe to evaluate the desired amount of great toe dorsiflexion.

Patients should be informed preoperatively that the rehabilitation protocol comprises marked restrictions for all physical activities during the first 6 weeks. Attributed to the surgeon's preference, postoperative ambulation includes a short leg cast, Lopresti slipper, or postoperative shoe. Furthermore, crutches may be necessary to reduce weight bearing on the concerned foot.

PLANNING THE OPERATION
Hallux Valgus et Rigidus

In patients with hallux valgus et rigidus deformity, the surgeon should take into consideration that MTP 1 joint arthrodesis reduces the first intermetatarsal angle up to 6°.[1,4,5] Therefore, an additional metatarsal osteotomy is not necessary for mild and moderate splayfoot deformities.

Lesser Toe Deformities

Concomitant lesser toe deformities have to be addressed simultaneously because intraoperative alignment of the great toe is closely related to the position of the adjacent toes. Therefore, it is mandatory to finish the realignment of the lesser toes before the MTP 1 joint is fixed with implants.

Central Metatarsalgia

Patients with hallux rigidus frequently complain of central metatarsalgia, which can be associated with calluses beneath the metatarsal heads. If the lesser toes present with sufficient ground contact and do not reveal any sagittal deformity, that is, dorsal subluxation, osteotomies of the lesser metatarsals are not required. It can be expected that MTP 1 joint arthrodesis regains normal load bearing of the first ray and subsequently reduces transfer metatarsalgia.

Toe Length

Preoperative planning should also focus on the length discrepancy between the great toe and the second toe. Regardless of the technique of cartilage debridement (flat cuts or cup and cone reamers), MTP 1 joint arthrodesis results in marked shortening (5–6 mm) of the great toe.[6] If a patient presents with a Greek foot (first toe<second toe), preoperative planning should include length balancing to avoid the onset of lesser toe deformity later. Length adjustment can be achieved by interposition of

a bone block at the MTP 1 joint or a shortening arthrodesis at the proximal interphalangeal joint of the second toe.

KEYSTONES OF THE SURGICAL PROCEDURE
Approach

Skin incision for MTP 1 joint arthrodesis can be performed at the medial side or the dorsal aspect of the MTP 1 joint. Because the type of incision has an effect on the joint exposure, the technique for cartilage debridement and fixation is determined by the approach. With a medial incision, only flat cuts can be made to resect the cartilage surfaces. Fixation is limited to screws or pins. The dorsal approach allows more technical alternatives, such as cup and cone reamers and dorsal plating.

Cartilage Debridement

The technique for cartilage resection is mainly determined by the bone quality. In patients with rheumatoid arthritis and osteoporosis, cartilage can be easily removed with a rongeur. This technique does not work in patients with hallux rigidus. Osteophytes and the sclerotic subchondral layer require high-speed instruments to remove the cartilage.

Flat cuts at the first metatarsal (MT 1) head and the proximal phalanx can be made with an oscillating saw.[7–9] Adjusting the saw blade is technically demanding because the surgeon has to consider both the transverse and the sagittal plane positions. Compared with the cup and cone technique, flat cuts have an increased potential for first ray shortening. To avoid this side effect, cartilage resection can be done with a crescentic saw blade.[10]

The cup and cone resection requires special power-driven instruments and a broad exposure of the joint with plantar dislocation of the great toe. Alignment of the reamers is facilitated by guide pins, which are inserted along the longitudinal axis of the proximal phalanx and the MT 1. Although cartilage removal at the metatarsal head is a simple and quick procedure, the preparation of the proximal phalanx is time consuming. Attributed to the sclerotic subchondral layer, the reamer has to be removed from the guide pin and cleaned several times. The anatomically shaped joint components allow intraoperative manipulation to achieve the optimal position of the great toe. Compared with flat cuts, the bone contact area is increased with the cup and cone technique,[11] which can be a theoretic advantage for bone healing. In the last few years, cup and cone reaming has gained wide popularity.[12–21]

Apart from the technique of cartilage debridement, multiple drilling of the subchondral layer (1.2–2.0 mm) is proposed to provoke subchondral bleeding and support bone healing.

Management of the Sesamoids

After circumferential debridement of the metatarsal head and the proximal phalanx, the sesamoids have to be assessed. Spurs and osteophytes at the sesamoids and the corresponding area of the MT 1 head and the proximal phalanx should be removed. Sometimes, it is also necessary to reshape and reduce the sesamoids in patients who present with enlarged and malformed sesamoids.

Alignment of the Great Toe

Three-plane positioning of the great toe must be adapted to the individual anatomic condition, level of activity, and shoe wear. Correct alignment of the great toe with sufficient ground contact is mandatory to assist balancing of the foot, assure physiologic load bearing of the forefoot, and prevent the IP 1 joint from degenerative changes.

In the transverse plane, 5° to 25° valgus is the desired position.[7,12,13,15–17,22–26] Apart from this recommendation, the great toe should be aligned parallel to the second toe, leaving a few millimeters space between the 2 toes.

Dorsiflexion of the great toe (sagittal plane) should be 10° to 15° in relation to the weight-bearing surface.[7,12,13,15–17,22–24,26,27] Compared with the MT 1, the weight-bearing surface is more reliable as a reference plane because it eliminates clinical variations, such as flatfoot, cavus foot, and declination of the MT 1.[12,16,17] Intraoperatively (patient in a supine position), the great toe alignment can be simulated by pressing a flat tray to the sole of the foot while the ankle is in neutral dorsiflexion. This simulation can greatly assist in assuring the appropriate positioning. The tip of the toe should stay approximately 5 mm from the tray surface.[28] Even in women who like to wear shoes with moderate heels, dorsiflexion of the MTP 1 joint should not exceed 15° because the dorsiflexed great toe may cause painful calluses at the IP 1 joint if patients wear comfortable shoes in between. A dorsiflexion of 15° allows one to wear shoes with a 2-in heel.[12]

In the frontal plane, the great toe should be aligned in neutral rotation, which can be easily calculated by the position of the nail.

Open Reduction Internal Fixation

Reliable internal fixation of the MTP 1 joint is a prerequisite to allow functional rehabilitation and to support bone healing.

Steinmann pins introduced longitudinally from the tip of the toe do not meet these requirements. Further disadvantages include hardware problems, lack of compression at the joint site, and damage to the IP 1 joint.

Even with 3 Kirschner wires (1 introduced longitudinally from the tip of the toe and 2 others crossing the joint), the stability is insufficient, so the failure rate (13.7%) is unacceptably high.[8]

Stabilization of the MTP 1 joint with simply a wire loop has also been reported as an inadequate fixation method with implant failure (26% wire breakage) and 38% nonunions.[29] Further biomechanical investigation revealed that the tension wire technique is 6 times weaker in load to failure than screw fixation.[30] Stability with the tension wire technique can be enhanced by introducing 2 separate loops (Ross-Smith technique, 1 loop in the transverse plane and 1 in the sagittal plane). Zafiropoulos and Henry[31] published a retrospective study of 48 patients (69 operations, arthrodesis with 2-loop stabilization), with a follow-up period of 6 years. Both reoperation rate (4%) and nonunions (4%) were low.

Use of staples for fixation of the MTP 1 joint arthrodesis is popular in France. Introduction of the implants is easy and time sparing. From a biomechanical point of view (stiffness and load to failure), staple use is clearly inferior to other methods, such as 2 crossed screws or dorsal plating.[32] Besse and coworkers[13] reported on 54 patients, with a follow-up period of 39 months. The investigators used 3 titanium staples to bridge the joint site. Clinical and radiological reviews showed 6% nonunions (2% reoperation rate). Choudhary and colleagues[23] used 2 Memory staples (Biopro Inc, Port Huron, MI, USA) to stabilize the MTP 1 joint and performed a prospective study on 27 patients (30 feet) with a follow-up period of 25 months. The investigators reported only 1 nonunion (3%), which has to be revised.

In the MTP 1 joint arthrodesis, screw fixation is the most frequently used method for stabilization. In 1952, McKeever[33] described the use of 1 screw, introduced plantarly through the proximal phalanx into the metatarsal shaft. Because of inherent rotational instability, the method is no longer in use.

Most surgeons use only 1 screw, placed from the medial side of the metatarsal head to the lateral cortex of the proximal phalanx. Wassink and van den Oever[9] analyzed 89 patients (109 feet) with a single screw stabilization technique. Nonunion occurred in 4.6%, and the technique had to be revised in all patients. In 78% of the patients, hardware problems made screw removal necessary.

Screw insertion can also be done from the distal medial aspect of the proximal phalanx to the lateral cortex of the metatarsal head. Agoropoulos and coworkers[34] presented a long-term retrospective study (42 patients; follow-up period, 21.5 years) with this method of stabilization. They reported only 1 patient with a bilateral nonunion (3.2%). Zafiropoulos and Henry,[31] on the other hand, could not confirm such encouraging results. In their study, 95 patients who underwent the single-screw technique were reanalyzed in a retrospectively controlled study after a mean follow-up period of 6 years. Of the 95 patients, 5.3% developed a nonunion, and the technique had to be revised. The total reoperation rate was 21% (6% malunions, 5% nonunions, 10% hardware problems).

Apart from the published results, it has to be considered that the use of a single screw has the potential risk of rotational instability, which may result in nonunion or malunion. This disadvantage can be overcome by using 2 screws. Turan and Lindgren[35] proposed to introduce 2 parallel screws from the medial side of the MT 1. This method has not gained popularity because of technical problems. Limited space at the lateral cortex of the proximal phalanx makes screw positioning difficult and often results in unintended phalanx fractures.

Using 2 crossed bicortical screws is one of the most popular fixation techniques to stabilize MTP 1 joint arthrodesis (**Fig. 1**). One screw runs from proximal medial to the lateral cortex of the proximal phalanx, whereas the other screw comes from the distal medial cortex and crosses the joint obliquely to the lateral aspect of the MT 1 head. To

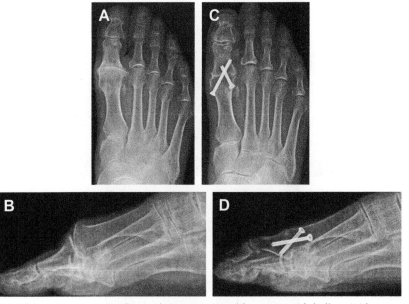

Fig. 1. (A) Anteroposterior radiograph in a 54-year-old woman with hallux rigidus stage 4. (B) Lateral radiograph showing marked elevation of the MT 1 with a plantar-flexed great toe. (C, D) Postoperative radiographs taken after a follow-up period of 6 months show solid bony fusion of the MTP 1 joint (2 crossed screws).

gain sufficient stability, the implants should cross each other within the distal region of the metatarsal head, not at the joint line. To avoid interference of the screws, it is recommended to introduce the first screw from plantar to dorsal and the second screw from dorsal to plantar. The use of cannulated screws facilitates positioning of the implants because the Kirschner wires give an idea of the second screw position. The reported nonunion rate after MTP 1 joint arthrodesis fixed with 2 crossed screws is 7.5%.[2,24,36,37] These case report studies refer to mixed indications (rheumatoid patients, revision surgery, hallux valgus) and various surgical techniques.

Isolated dorsal plating has a limited effect on interfragmentary compression **(Fig. 2)**. Retrospective studies revealed a mean nonunion rate of 9.9% with a singular dorsal plate.[11,20,36] Therefore, the dorsal plating should be combined with an interfragmentary screw. From a biomechanical point of view, this combination is twice as strong as 2 crossed screws.[38,39] For this reason, it is not surprising that the reported nonunion rates are low (3.9%).[7,19–21]

Summarizing the information on various internal fixation methods for MTP 1 joint arthrodesis revealed clear advantages for the dorsal plating combined with an interfragmentary screw.

New Techniques

It is obvious that percutaneous techniques have gained popularity. Bauer and coworkers[27] presented their surgical technique. Besides a standard medial approach, accessory portals can be added to remove osteophytes or to perform a lateral release.

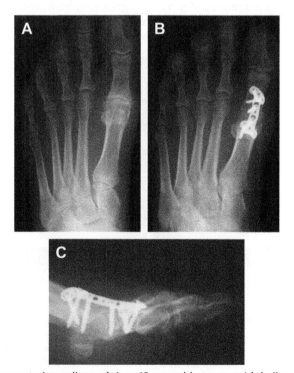

Fig. 2. (A) Anteroposterior radiograph in a 48-year-old woman with hallux rigidus stage 3. (B, C) Postoperative radiographs taken after a follow-up period of 6 months show solid bony fusion of the MTP 1 joint (dorsal plate).

Cartilage removal can be done with conical reamers creating flat bony surfaces. The investigators retrospectively reviewed the patients (n = 32) after a mean follow-up period of 18 months. The American Orthopaedic Foot and Ankle Society score improved significantly from 36 points preoperatively to 80 points at follow-up. Complications included 1 nonunion and 1 infection.

Complications

Malalignment of the great toe can cause painful callosities and transfer metatarsalgia. Too much dorsiflexion results in limited loading of the great toe and flexion at the IP 1 joint as an attempt to reach the ground. The dorsiflexed great toe makes shoe fitting difficult because the dorsal aspect of the toe impinges within the shoe. Overload of the MT 1 head can also occur because the great toe does not respond to sufficient load bearing. If conservative measures (insole) fail, revision (osteotomy) is indicated.

Too much plantar flexion of the great toe may cause abutment and pressure to the great toe. Walking mainly affects the IP 1 joint, which is passively dorsiflexed during toe-off. This repetitive stress can lead to painful joint degeneration. To reduce pain, patients can be advised to wear rocker bottom shoes.

Frontal plane malalignment is a rare finding. If malrotation had occurred, patients mostly complain of painful calluses at the condyles of the distal phalanx.

A valgus position of the great toe can present with painful impinging of the second toe. Before any surgical suggestions, it should be assessed if the transversal malalignment is caused by a hallux valgus interphalangeus or a true hallux valgus deformity from the MTP 1 joint. Conservative measures are limited to soft pads placed in the first web space. If surgical revision is indicated, the site of osteotomy should refer to the underlying pathologic condition of malalignment.

Hallux varus deformity exceeding 10° can lead to shoe wear problems, if the great toe impinges against the shoe. Patients are advised to wear shoes with a broad toe box and soft leather. Otherwise, the great toe has to be realigned by an osteotomy.

Nonunion is a typical complication after MTP 1 joint arthrodesis that can even occur after meticulous cartilage debridement and sufficient internal fixation. It is obvious that patients with a fibrous nonunion can be asymptomatic. Therefore, revision surgery (debridement, bone grafting) is indicated only in case of painful nonunions.

Results

The clinical results after arthrodesis of the MTP 1 joint (**Table 1**) are strictly related to the surgical technique and the device used for internal fixation. Because most articles[11,18,19,21,25,40–42] refer to mixed indications (hallux rigidus, hallux valgus, rheumatoid patients, revision surgery), the evaluation and rating of any surgical management becomes difficult. In summarizing the most representative studies, these restraints should be considered.

Personal Technique

With the patient in a supine position, a thigh tourniquet is applied. Using a dorsal incision, the extensor hood is incised medial to the extensor hallucis tendon. In patients with additional hallux valgus, the extensor hood is incised laterally.

The exposed joint comprises 2 full thickness capsular flaps. The MT 1 head and the proximal phalanx are exposed circumferentially to remove the osteophytes even at the sesamoids.

Cartilage debridement is mainly done with concave/convex reamers to attain an appropriate shape. Additional drilling of both the joint components is routinely performed to perforate the subchondral layer.

Table 1
Clinical results after arthrodesis of the MTP 1 joint from several studies

References	Study Design	Number of Patients	Follow-up (mo)	AOFAS Forefoot Score (Preoperative/Postoperative)	Nonunion (%)	Revision (%)
Lombardi et al,[40] 2001	Retrospective	21	28	39/76	14.3	19
Coughlin & Shurnas,[41] 2004	Retrospective	34	80	38/89	5.8	0
Aslam & Ribbans,[18] 2005	Retrospective	33	28	44/82	3	9
Goucher & Coughlin,[11] 2006	Prospective	53	16	51/82	8	4
Beertema et al,[25] 2006	Retrospective	34	84	?/78	11.7	12
Raikin et al,[42] 2007	Retrospective	27	30	36/84	3.7	0
Bennett & Sabetta,[21] 2009	Prospective	200	?	41/84	1.3	1.3
Kumar et al,[19] 2010	Retrospective	46	23	?/82	2.1	2.1

Abbreviations: AOFAS, American Orthopaedic Foot and Ankle Society; ?, no data provided in original source.

The great toe is then aligned parallel to the second toe with some space between the toes. To get an impression of the great toe's dorsiflexion, a flat tray is pressed to the sole of the foot, with the ankle in neutral position. The great toe should either be less than 5 mm away from the tray or somewhat touch the tray. The desired position is temporarily fixed with a Kirschner wire to allow fluoroscopic imaging.

The first interfragmentary screw (3.5–4.0 mm) is inserted from the proximal medial aspect of the MT 1 head toward the suprabasal lateral aspect of the proximal phalanx. The screw must penetrate the lateral cortex to achieve sufficient interfragmentary compression. After medial eminence resection, the soft spongious bone sometimes does not sufficiently buttress the head of the screw, which may uneventfully countersink into the bone. In such instances, the screw should be inserted from a more proximal position (stab incision) to attain sufficient cortical support.

A contoured locking plate with an appropriate length (at least 2 screws in the proximal phalanx) is placed dorsally and temporarily fixed with Kirschner wires. The plate should display an appropriate fit to the dorsal cortex. The length of the screws is checked fluoroscopically to avoid interference with the sesamoids proximally.

After fluoroscopic controls, the wound is closed in layers followed by a bulky compressive dressing. Patients are advised to elevate the foot and limit walking during the first 3 days. Although patients can ambulate with full weight bearing in a postoperative shoe, use of crutches is proposed to reduce pain during the first week.

Radiographic imaging is performed after 6 weeks. If sufficient bone healing has occurred, patients are allowed to wear rocker bottom shoes with a stiff sole for another 6 weeks. The final clinical and radiological control takes place after 12 weeks (**Fig. 3**).

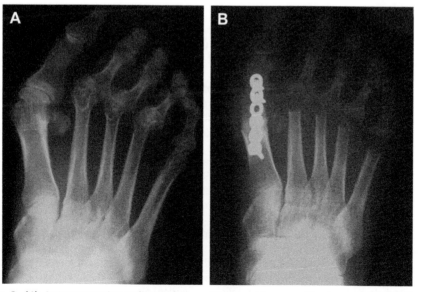

Fig. 3. (*A*) Anteroposterior radiograph in a 67-year-old man with rheumatoid forefoot deformity with painful MTP joints. (*B*) Postoperative radiograph taken after a follow-up period of 3 months shows solid fusion of the MTP 1 joint (dorsal plate) and lesser metatarsal head resection.

SUMMARY

Arthrodesis of the MTP 1 joint is the method of choice for end-stage painful joint degeneration. It can be drawn from the literature that the technique for cartilage debridement and the internal fixation method mainly influence the outcome. Despite the fusion of a key joint, there is little adverse effect on gait, and weight bearing of the first ray can be restored.

REFERENCES

1. Lombardi C, Silhanek A, Connolly F, et al. The effect of first metatarsophalangeal joint arthrodesis on the first ray and the medial longitudinal arch: a radiographic study. J Foot Ankle Surg 2002;41:96–103.
2. Brodsky JW, Baum BS, Pollo FE, et al. Prospective gait analysis in patients with first metatarsophalangeal joint arthrodesis for hallux rigidus. Foot Ankle Int 2007;28:162–5.
3. De Frino PF, Brodsky JW, Pollo FE, et al. First metatarsophalangeal arthrodesis: a clinical, pedobarographic and gait analysis study. Foot Ankle Int 2002;23: 496–502.
4. Humbert JL, Bourbonnière C, Laurin CA. Metatarsophalangeal fusion for hallux valgus: indications and effects on the first metatarsal ray. Can Med Assoc J 1979;120:937.
5. Sung W, Kluesner AJ, Irrgang J, et al. Radiographic outcomes following primary arthrodesis of the first metatarsophalangeal joint in hallux abductovalgus deformity. J Foot Ankle Surg 2010;49:446–51.
6. Singh B, Draeger R, Del Gaizo GJ, et al. Changes in length of the first ray with two different first MTP fusion techniques: a cadaveric study. Foot Ankle Int 2008;29: 722–5.
7. Sharma H, Bhagat S, Deleeuw J, et al. In vivo comparison of screw versus plate and screw fixation for first metatarsophalangeal arthrodesis: does augmentation of internal compression screw fixation using a semi-tubular plate shorten time to clinical and radiologic fusion of the first metatarsophalangeal joint (MTPJ)? J Foot Ankle Surg 2008;47:2–7.
8. Mah CD, Banks AS. Immediate weight bearing following first metatarsophalangeal joint fusion with Kirschner wire fixation. J Foot Ankle Surg 2009;48:3–8.
9. Wassink S, van den Oever M. Arthrodesis of the first metatarsophalangeal joint using a single screw: retrospective analysis of 109 feet. J Foot Ankle Surg 2009;48:653–61.
10. Shute GC, Sferra JJ. Use of the crescentic saw for arthrodesis of the first metatarsophalangeal joint. Foot Ankle Int 1998;19:719–20.
11. Goucher NR, Coughlin MJ. Hallux metatarsophalangeal joint arthrodesis using dome shaped reamers and dorsal plate fixation: a prospective study. Foot Ankle Int 2006;27:869–76.
12. Kelikian AS. Technical considerations in hallux metatarsophalangeal arthrodesis. Foot Ankle Clin 2005;10:167–90.
13. Besse JL, Chouteau J, Laptoiu D. Arthrodesis of the first metatarsophalangeal joint with ball and cup reamers and osteosynthesis with pure titanium staples. Radiological evaluation of a continuous series of 54 cases. Foot Ankle Surg 2010;16:32–7.
14. Patel A, Baumhauer J. First metatarsophalangeal joint arthrodesis. Operat Tech Orthop 2008;18:216–20.

15. Aas M, Johnsen TM, Finsen V. Arthrodesis of the first metatarsophalangeal joint for hallux rigidus—optimal position of fusion. Foot (Edinb) 2008;18:131–5.
16. Womack JW, Ishikawa SN. First metatarsophalangeal arthrodesis. Foot Ankle Clin N Am 2009;14:43–50.
17. Hamilton GA, Ford LA, Patel S. First metatarsophalangeal joint arthrodesis and revision arthrodesis. Clin Podiatr Med Surg 2009;26:459–73.
18. Aslam N, Ribbans WJ. First metatarsophalangeal joint arthrodesis using a vitallium plate with a mean two year follow up. Foot Ankle Surg 2005;11: 197–201.
19. Kumar S, Pradhan R, Rosenfeld PF. First metatarsophalangeal arthrodesis using a dorsal plate and a compression screw. Foot Ankle Int 2010;31:797–801.
20. Ellington JK, Jones CP, Cohen BE, et al. Review of 107 hallux MTP joint arthrodesis using dome-shaped reamers and a stainless-steel dorsal plate. Foot Ankle Int 2010;31:385–90.
21. Bennett GL, Sabetta J. First metatarsophalangeal joint arthrodesis: evaluation of plate and screw fixation. Foot Ankle Int 2009;30:752–7.
22. Fadel GE, Rowley DI, Abboud RJ. Hallux metatarsophalangeal joint arthrodesis: various techniques. The Foot 2002;12:88–96.
23. Choudhary RK, Theruvil B, Taylor GR. First metatarsophalangeal joint arthrodesis: a new technique of internal fixation by using memory compression staples. J Foot Ankle Surg 2004;43:312–7.
24. Gröndal L, Stark A. Fusion of the first metatarsophalangeal joint, a review of techniques and considerations. Presentation of our results in 22 cases. The Foot 2005;15:86–90.
25. Beertema W, Draijer WF, van Os JJ, et al. A retrospective analysis of surgical treatment in patients with symptomatic hallux rigidus: long-term follow-up. J Foot Ankle Surg 2006;45:244–51.
26. Alexander P, Lau J. First metatarsophalangeal arthrodesis. Operat Tech Orthop 2009;19:221–5.
27. Bauer T, Lortat-Jacob A, Hardy P. First metatarsophalangeal joint percutaneous arthrodesis. Orthop Traumatol Surg Res 2010;96:567–73.
28. Harper MC. Positioning of the hallux for first metatarsalphalangeal joint arthrodesis. Foot Ankle Int 1997;18:827.
29. Shahane SA, Vedantam R, Bhadreshwar DR. Arthrodesis of the first metatarsophalangeal joint using AO tension band wire. The Foot 1995;5:15–8.
30. Faraj AA, Naraen A, Twigg P. A comparative study of wire fixation and screw fixation in arthrodesis for the correction of hallux rigidus using an in vitro biomechanical model. Foot Ankle Int 2007;28:89–91.
31. Zafiropoulos G, Henry APJ. Comparison study of two methods of fusion of the first metatarsophalangeal joint. The Foot 1994;4:59–61.
32. Neufeld SK, Parks BG, Naseef GS, et al. Arthrodesis of the first metatarsophalangeal joint: a biomechanical study comparing memory compression staples, cannulated screws, and a dorsal plate. Foot Ankle Int 2002;23:97–101.
33. McKeever DC. Arthrodesis of the first metatarsophalangeal joint for hallux valgus, hallux rigidus, and metatarsus primus varus. J Bone Joint Surg Am 1952;34: 129–34.
34. Agoropoulos Z, Efsthathopoulos N, Mataliotakis J, et al. Long-term results of first metatarsophalangeal joint fusion for severe hallux valgus deformity. Foot Ankle Surg 2001;7:9–13.
35. Turan I, Lindgren U. Compression-screw arthrodesis of the first metatarsophalangeal joint of the foot. Clin Orthop 1987;221:292–5.

36. Hyer CF, Glover JP, Berlet GC, et al. Cost comparison of crossed screws versus dorsal plate construct for first metatarsophalangeal joint arthrodesis. J Foot Ankle Surg 2008;47:13–8.
37. Jardé O, Laya Z, Olory B, et al. Arthrodesis of the first metatarsophalangeal joint using convex and concave drills: a report on 50 cases. Acta Orthop Belg 2005;71:76–82.
38. Politi J, John H, Njus G, et al. First metatarsal-phalangeal joint arthrodesis: a biomechanical assessment of stability. Foot Ankle Int 2003;24:332–7.
39. Buranosky DJ, Taylor DT, Sage RA, et al. First metatarsophalangeal joint arthrodesis: quantitative mechanical testing of six hole dorsal plate versus crossed screw fixation in cadaveric specimens. J Foot Ankle Surg 2001;40:208–13.
40. Lombardi CM, Silhanek AD, Connolly FG, et al. First metatarsophalangeal arthrodesis for treatment of hallux rigidus: a retrospective study. J Foot Ankle Surg 2001;40:137–43.
41. Coughlin MJ, Shurnas PS. Hallux rigidus: grading and long-term results of operative treatment. J Bone Joint Surg Am 2004;85:2072–88.
42. Raikin SM, Ahmad J, Pour AE, et al. Comparison of arthrodesis and metallic hemiarthroplasty of the hallux metatarsophalangeal joint. J Bone Joint Surg Am 2007;89(9):1979–85.

First Metatarsophalangeal Arthrodesis for Severe Bone Loss

Reinhard Schuh, MD[a,b], Hans-Joerg Trnka, MD[a,*]

KEYWORDS

- Metatarsophalangeal joint • Arthrodesis • Bone loss
- Hallux valgus

Severe bone loss of the first metatarsal is a challenging problem for foot and ankle surgeons. The bone loss of the first metatarsophalangeal (MTP) joint may be related to an infection, rheumatoid arthritis–related destruction, and in most cases iatrogenic because of previous hallux valgus or hallux rigidus surgery. Numerous procedures for hallux valgus and rigidus correction have been proposed in the literature, causing various complications, such as hallux varus, first MTP joint instability, infection, recurrent hallux valgus, and avascular necrosis (AVN). A first MTP joint arthrodesis is often the method of choice to salvage this situation.[1–3]

With minimal to moderate bone loss, hallux MTP joint arthrodesis is performed in situ, accepting a slight shortening of the hallux. In the authors' opinion, the slight shortening creates minimal cosmetic concerns and affords satisfactory functional improvement in most cases. Furthermore, the morbidity and risk of complications after in situ fusion is less than after bone block distraction fusion.

When previous surgeries have led to bone loss and shortening of the proximal phalanx or first metatarsal, especially in cases after failed joint implants, prior resection arthroplasty (such as the Keller-type arthroplasty), and revision arthrodesis for healed malunions or nonunions, it is necessary to restore the length of the great toe (**Figs. 1** and **2**).[4] Significant changes of the length of the first ray have a clinical significance, as the first ray, along with the fifth ray and the calcaneus, forms a tripod for weight bearing. Changes in the length of the first ray can cause critical alterations in the biomechanics of the foot, which could potentially allow for partial weight-bearing points of contact.[5] The first ray has been found to support at least one-third of the

[a] Foot and Ankle Center Vienna, Alserstrasse 43/8D, 1080 Vienna, Austria
[b] Department of Orthopaedic Surgery, Innsbruck Medical University, Anichstrasse 35, 6020 Innsbruck, Austria
* Corresponding author.
E-mail address: trnka@fusszentrum.at

Foot Ankle Clin N Am 16 (2011) 13–20
doi:10.1016/j.fcl.2010.11.005
1083-7515/11/$ – see front matter © 2011 Published by Elsevier Inc.

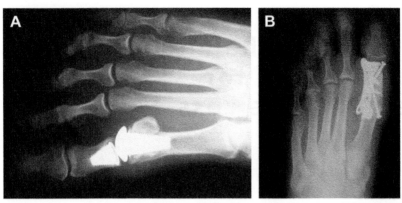

Fig. 1. (*A*) Anteroposterior radiograph of a patient with failed first MTP joint arthroplasty caused by implant malposition. (*B*) A bone block fusion was performed as salvage procedure.

forefoot weight during the stance phase of gait.[6] Furthermore, approximately 40% to 60% of the body weight passes through the first MTP joint and great toe during normal gait.[7] During athletic activities, these forces can approach 2 to 3 times the body weight, especially with jogging and running.[8]

With marked shortening of the hallux and associated lesser metatarsalgia, an in situ hallux MTP joint arthrodesis may fail to restore satisfactory function. An interpositional structural bone graft from the iliac crest is used to restore first ray length, which, in turn, should improve the weight bearing of the first metatarsal and hallux while alleviating lesser metatarsalgia. An interpositional bone graft can accomplish the goals of restoring length and filling defects in the native bone, but making accurate flat surface cuts and achieving proper fusion may be technically difficult.[9–11] A cup-in-cone

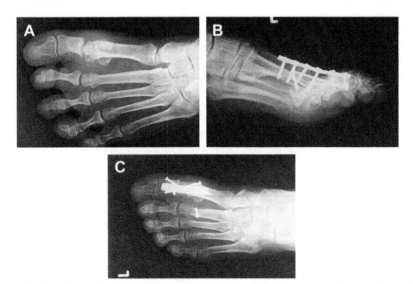

Fig. 2. (*A–C*) Radiographs of a patient after Mayo procedure. Because of severe bone loss, a bone block arthrodesis was performed.

reamer used for contouring the interpositional graft may help to provide proper thickness of the graft to gain length of the great toe.[4]

Sources for structural interposition bone block arthrodesis include the following:

1. Structural allograft (usually contoured from a donor femoral head or iliac crest) or
2. Structural autograft (typically obtained from the patient's iliac crest or lateral aspect of the calcaneus).

Ipsilateral anterior iliac crest harvesting is ideal for foot and ankle surgery because this site is readily accessible in the patient positioned supine on the operating table.

Several methods have been described for contouring the interpositional graft. The authors' method of choice is the ball-and-socket technique, which affords 3 advantages over flat cuts or a conical preparation.

PATIENT HISTORY

The patient's major complaint is pain in the first MTP joint region and/or at the lateral aspect of the forefoot caused by pathologic force distribution during the stance phase of gait (lateralization of center of pressure). The patient's history includes failed primary hallux valgus surgery (especially in cases of previous resectional arthroplasties) or failed primary MTP fusion and total joint alloarthroplasty.[12]

The physical examination should include assessment of the neurovascular status, hallux position, shortening of the first ray, range of motion of the first interphalangeal (IP) joint, and pain and crepitus with range of motion of the hallux. Forefoot pronation and supination with regards to the first ray should be noted.[13] Instrumented examinations like the dynamic plantar pressure analysis could be used to objectively assess abnormalities of the stance phase of gait. In addition, the site of bone graft harvesting (iliac crest, lateral aspect of the calcaneus, proximal tibia) should be inspected for unanticipated soft tissue concerns.

NONOPERATIVE TREATMENT

Nonoperative treatment options include the use of forefoot support provided by custom-made insoles to unload the lesser metatarsal heads. However, for the severely shortened first ray, this treatment option might often be insufficient.

PREOPERATIVE PLANNING

Weight-bearing anteroposterior (AP)- and lateral-view radiographs are taken. In case of residual hallux valgus deformity, the hallux valgus angle and intermetatarsal angle should be assessed in the AP plane. An external oblique view can add information about the amount of the osseous defect.[13] In addition, magnetic resonance imaging of the forefoot might be useful to assess the amount of necrotic bone in cases of AVN of the first metatarsal head.

Preoperatively, it has to be decided if a structural femoral head of iliac crest allograft or an iliac crest autograft will be taken. Both procedures have specific advantages and disadvantages. Theoretically, there is the possibility of transmission of disease and malignancy when using a structural allograft. However, Myerson and colleagues[14] reported no case of transmission of disease in an investigation of structural allografts for foot and ankle surgery. The risk of autologous iliac bone graft is donor site morbidity, including local hematoma, local infection, and local nerve irritation.[15]

A preoperative drawing may help to determine the approximate amount of bone resection and the length of the graft that is required.

SURGICAL TECHNIQUE

The patient is placed in the supine position on the operating table. The procedure should be performed without a tourniquet to assess the vitality of the bone intraoperatively.

Regardless of existing scars, a standard dorsal approach is recommended. This approach allows adequate exposure of the MTP joint and avoids damage of the medial dorsal cutaneous nerve, which is difficult to identify in the scar tissue.[16] The skin incision starts about 4 cm proximal to the first MTP joint and extends to the first IP joint (**Fig. 3**). Depending on the amount of shortening and presence of cock-up deformity, the flexor hallucis longus tendon is retracted laterally or cut in a Z shape to facilitate exposure to the MTP joint. In case of cock-up deformity, it is necessary to lengthen this tendon.

The joint capsule and the soft tissue coverage of the metatarsal and the phalanx are incised longitudinally straight down to the bone and then opened as an envelope. Subperiosteal preparation is mandatory to ensure sufficient release from the lateral soft tissue and scar adhesions. Only the plantar aspect is left intact to preserve the blood supply to both bones. Osteophytes and remaining soft tissue adhesions are removed at this point. After this, the big toe is brought into maximal plantarflexion.

If a cup-in-cone reamer is used for the preparation of joint surfaces and removal of remaining cartilage tissue, a guidewire has to be inserted in the center of the metatarsal head. A ball-in-socket preparation provides the advantage of minimizing bone loss and creates the ability to alter the position of the toe after the preparation has been performed. Basically, it can be performed with spherical reamers, chisels, or a rongeur. After inserting the guidewire, the appropriately sized "female" reamer is placed over the guidewire. The reaming is performed until cancellous bleeding bone can be visualized. Then, the proximal phalanx is exposed, and a guidewire is placed in the center of the articular surface area. The "male" reamer counterpart is placed over the guidewire, and the surface is prepared in the aforementioned manner.

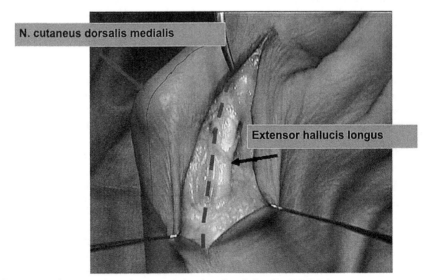

N. cutaneus dorsalis medialis

Extensor hallucis longus

Fig. 3. Dorsal approach and anatomic landmarks of the first MTP joint.

Now, the toe can be pulled into the position of desired length, and the exact extent of the gap in the joint is measured.

The skin incision at the iliac crest is centered 3 cm posterior to the anterior superior iliac spine. The preparation of the soft tissue is performed using electrocautery for hemostasis until the periostium of the superior crest is reached. Two Hohmann retractors are introduced, and the desired segment for harvesting is marked. The length is determined by the gap created with the first MTP joint preparation. At this stage, a saw is used to osteomize the ends of the tricortical bone block. The autogenous graft is harvested, and the defect may be backfilled with allograft bone chips. After drain placement, the periostium is closed and wound closure is performed in a common manner.[15]

The graft (either autogenous or allogenous) should be secured on the back table using a forceps to be shaped into the desired length. A guidewire for the cup-in-cone reamer set is placed in the center of the graft's longitudinal axis. The graft margins are marked, and the graft ends are contoured with the reamers. Two corresponding ends are prepared to create optimal contact to the host bone (**Fig. 4**).

The molded graft is inserted in the gap between the proximal phalanx and the first metatarsal. Either a standard plate or a special revision plate is placed dorsally, and temporary fixation of the construct is performed using pins. The position of the arthrodesis is crucial. Excessive plantarflexion or dorsiflexion has to be avoided. Therefore, the lid of an instrument tray can be used to simulate the floor with weight bearing. A correct position in the sagittal plane is obtained when the tip of the toe (distal phalanx) is able to exert pressure on the ground when the patient is standing. In general, a dorsiflexion angle of 20° to 25° between the metatarsal and the phalanx

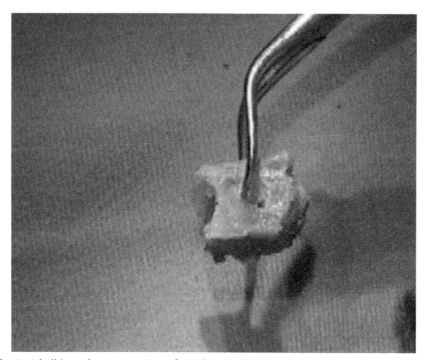

Fig. 4. A ball-in-socket preparation of autologous iliac crest bone graft.

is recommended, but the individual first metatarsal inclination angle has to be considered.[17] Excessive dorsiflexion may cause overload of the sesamoids, symptomatic irritation of the hallux in shoe, and poor cosmetic appearance, whereas excessive plantarflexion leads to symptoms during push off in the stance phase of gait and eventually to IP joint arthrosis. A varus position makes wearing shoes difficult; an excessive valgus position impinges the second toe. Therefore, a neutral to slight valgus position is recommended.

For fixation of the arthrodesis, a 3.0-mm or 3.5-mm cannulated screw is inserted from the medial aspect of the residual proximal phalanx across the graft to the lateral aspect of the residual metatarsal. The plate is secured to the construct with screws in the proximal phalanx, graft, and metatarsal. All the fixation processes are performed under fluoroscopic guidance.

A small-diameter drain is introduced, and closure of the wound is performed in a proper manner.

POSTOPERATIVE REGIMEN

Sterile dressings are applied to the wound, and the foot is placed for a total of 6 to 8 weeks in a short-leg cast that extends beyond the toes. Non–weight bearing is recommended until suture removal 2 weeks postoperatively, after which partial weight bearing until 6 to 8 weeks should be performed.

Full weight bearing can be anticipated when there is radiographic evidence of bony fusion.

RESULTS

In a retrospective study, Myerson and colleagues[10] investigated 24 patients who underwent first MTP joint arthrodesis using bone graft to restore length. All patients underwent previous surgery for correction of hallux valgus deformity or hallux rigidus, which resulted in significant bone loss. The clinical and radiographic follow-up was performed at an average of 62.7 months after surgery. In 79.1% of the patients, successful fusion was noted at a mean of 13.3 weeks after surgery and the first ray was lengthened by a mean of 13 mm. There were a total of 5 nonunions; 3 of them were symptomatic and successfully managed with further surgery. In this series, 1 deep infection and 2 superficial infections were reported. The mean American Orthopaedic Foot and Ankle Society (AOFAS) score improved from 39 points preoperatively to 79 points at follow-up.

Another study by Brodsky and colleagues[11] investigated 12 patients with salvaged first MTP arthrodesis with structural interpositional autologous iliac crest bone graft. Indication for surgery was severe bone loss after MTP joint alloplasties in 8 patients, AVN after failed hallux valgus surgery in 2 patients, nonunion after primary MTP arthrodesis in 1 patient and osteomyelitis after cheilectomy in 1 patient. The graft was augmented with a single dorsal plate in 11 cases and a dorsal and medial plate in 1 patient. At a mean of 15 weeks, arthrodesis was achieved in 11 of 12 cases. The nonunion was asymptomatic and did not need further treatment. The AOFAS score averaged 70 points at 22 months follow-up. Two cases required flap coverage for skin necrosis.

Vienne and colleagues[18] stated that the AOFAS score increased from 44 to 85 at an average follow-up of 34 months in 20 patients who underwent MTP joint arthrodesis after failed Keller-Brandes procedure. However, most patients of this study had in situ fusion and did not require interpositional bone graft. Assessment of dynamic plantar pressure distribution of these patients revealed that, biomechanically, the

MTP joint arthrodesis could not fully restore the function of the hallux but produced a significant improvement, allowing a more physiologic loading pattern under the hallux and the metatarsal head.

SUMMARY

Studies have demonstrated that shortening of the first ray can lead to symptomatic forefoot disorders, such as transfer metatarsalgia of the lesser toes.[7,19] Therefore, in cases of MTP arthrodesis, care has to be taken to avoid shortening of the first ray. In case of revisional arthrodesis with severe bone loss, interpositional bone block arthrodesis is a reliable procedure that results in good clinical and functional results.

REFERENCES

1. Trnka HJ. Arthrodesis procedures for salvage of the hallux metatarsophalangeal joint. Foot Ankle Clin 2000;5(3):673–86.
2. Myerson M, Miller SD, Henderson MR, et al. Staged arthrodesis for salvage of the septic hallux metatarsophalangeal joint. Clin Orthop Relat Res 1994;307:174–81.
3. Coughlin MJ, Mann RA. Arthrodesis of the first metatarsophalangeal joint as salvage for the failed Keller procedure. J Bone Joint Surg Am 1987;69:68–75.
4. Whalen J. Clinical tip: interpositional bone graft for first MP fusion. Foot Ankle Int 2009;30(2):160–2.
5. Singh B, Draeger R, Del Gaizo DJ, et al. Changes in length of the first ray with two different first MTP fusion techniques: a cadaveric study. Foot Ankle Int 2008; 29(7):722–5.
6. Sammarco G. Biomechanics of the foot. Philadelphia: Lea & Febiger; 1980. p. 123–220.
7. Stokes IA, Hutton WC, Stott JR, et al. Forces under the hallux valgus foot before and after surgery. Clin Orthop Relat Res 1979;142:64–72.
8. Nigg B. Biomechanical aspects of running. Champaign (IL): Human Kinetics; 1986. p. 1–25.
9. Goucher M, Coughlin MJ. Hallux metatarsophalangeal arthrodesis using dome-shaped reamers and dorsal plate fixation. A prospective study. Foot Ankle Int 2006;27:869–76.
10. Myerson M, Schon LC, McGuigan FX, et al. Results of arthrodesis of the hallux metatarsophalangeal joint using bone graft for restoration of length. Foot Ankle Int 2000;21:297–306.
11. Brodsky JW, Ptaszek AJ, Morris SG. Salvage first MTP arthrodesis utilizing ICBG: clinical evaluation and outcome. Foot Ankle Int 2000;21:290–6.
12. Machacek F Jr, Easley ME, Gruber F, et al. Salvage of failed Keller resection arthroplasty. J Bone Joint Surg Am 2004;86:1131–8.
13. Kelikian AS. Technical considerations in metatarsophalangeal joint arthrodesis. Foot Ankle Clin 2005;10:167–90.
14. Myerson M, Neufeld SK, Uribe J. Fresh frozen structural allografts in the foot and ankle. J Bone Joint Surg Am 2005;87 A:113–20.
15. Hofstaetter S, Trnka HJ. Bone block distraction for the first metatarsophalangeal joint. In: Easley ME, Weisel SW, editors. Operative techniques in foot and ankle surgery (Operative techniques in orthopaedic surgery). Philadelphia (PA): Lippincott Williams & Wilkins; 2010. p. 1–9.
16. Machacek F Jr, Easley ME, Gruber F, et al. Salvage of the failed Keller resection arthroplasty. Surgical technique. J Bone Joint Surg Am 2005;87(Suppl 1[Pt 1]): 86–94.

17. Bayomy AF, Aubin PM, Sangeorzan BJ, et al. Arthrodesis of the first metatarso-phalangeal joint: a robotic cadaver study of the dorsiflexion angle. J Bone Joint Surg Am 2010;92:1754–64.
18. Vienne P, Sukthankar A, Favre Ph, et al. Metatarsophalangeal joint arthrodesis after failed Keller-Brandes procedure. Foot Ankle Int 2006;27(11):894–901.
19. Waldecker U. Metatarsalgia in hallux valgus deformity: a pedographic analysis. J Foot Ankle Surg 2002;41(5):300–8.

Tarsometatarsal Arthrodesis for Management of Unstable First Ray and Failed Bunion Surgery

Norman Espinosa, MD*, Stephan H. Wirth, MD

KEYWORDS

• Tarsometatarsal • Arthrodesis • Hypermobility • First ray
• Hallux valgus

Historically, the first metatarsocuneiform joint has been recognized as a source of forefoot abnormality. Morton[1] believed that hypermobility of the first ray led to abnormal load transfer to the lesser metatarsals and the combination of a short first metatarsal and hypermobility of the first ray was responsible for major dysfunction at the forefoot. Courriades[2] defined hypermobility of the first ray as a separate clinical entity. Lapidus,[3] who suggested fusion to correct the pathologic condition, made similar observations on the first ray. Although Lapidus became famous for having popularized the closing wedge arthrodesis of the first metatarsocuneiform joint, it was Albrecht who, in 1911, first described this kind of procedure to treat hallux valgus associated with metatarsus primus varus. Other investigators, such as Truslow[4] (1925) and Kleinberg[5] (1932), followed Albrecht and published their reports on similar operations long before Lapidus did. The fusion of the first metatarsocuneiform joint, that is, the first tarsometatarsal joint (TMT-1), provides a reliable means for the management of many forefoot abnormalities, including failed bunion surgery and hallux valgus correction in the presence of first ray hypermobility. The latter remains a subject of ongoing research. During the last 2 decades, significant advances have been made to understand hypermobility of the first ray. However, the exact role in the development of hallux valgus is yet to be determined.

The authors have nothing to disclose.
Department of Orthopaedics, University of Zurich, Balgrist, Forchstrasse 340, 8008 Zurich, Switzerland
* Corresponding author.
E-mail address: norman.espinosa@balgrist.ch

ANATOMY OF THE TMT-1

The joints formed by the bases of the metatarsal bones and the 3 cuneiforms are known as the Lisfranc joint.[6,7] At their proximal site, the bases of the 5 metatarsals are arranged in an arcuate fashion, the second metatarsal base being the apex of the mediolateral arch of the midfoot. The inclinations of the metatarsal shafts contribute to the longitudinal arch of the foot, which is more pronounced on the medial than on the lateral side. The first metatarsal bone is either shorter or of equal length when compared with the second metatarsal bone.[8] The medial cuneiform and the base of the first metatarsal are slightly obliquely orientated toward the medial metatarsal. In addition, the first metatarsal bone diverges slightly from the second metatarsal bone. The normal 1–2 intermetatarsal angle in adults has been found to range between 3° to 9°.[9] In the sagittal plane, the joint orientation is from dorsal distal to plantar proximal. This inclination allows the first metatarsal base to support the medial cuneiform. The medial cuneiform has a convex medial border and a concave lateral border. The base of the first metatarsal bone comprises 3 articular surfaces that articulate with the surface of the medial cuneiform. At the junction of the medial and inferior surfaces is a small tubercle that provides an insertion site for the anterior tibial tendon. The peroneus longus tendon inserts at a more pronounced tubercle at the junction of the inferior and lateral surfaces of the base of the first metatarsal. There is no ligamentous connection between the first and second metatarsal bases. The joint is stabilized on the medial side by a dorsal cuneometatarsal ligament and on the lateral side by the plantar cuneometatarsal ligaments. The strongest ligament is arranged in a more dorsomedial fashion and contributes to the capsule of the TMT-1. A more rectangular plantar ligament connects the base of the first metatarsal to the cuneiform. Mizel[10] demonstrated that the first plantar cuneometatarsal ligament is the key to resisting dorsal displacement of the first ray. The Lisfranc ligament runs plantarly between the medial cuneiform and the base of the second and third metatarsals. It is considered a key ligament and stabilizes the medial to the intermediate and lateral column.[11]

BIOMECHANICS OF THE FIRST METATARSOCUNEIFORM JOINT

First ray stability depends on both structural and dynamic support. Structural support is provided by the bony and ligamentous architecture of the midfoot. Normally, the joints between the bases of the metatarsals and 3 cuneiforms only provide little motion. The joints are intrinsically stable because of their archlike and interdigitating configuration. The second metatarsal base is recessed into the mortise formed at the midfoot between the base of the first metatarsal, medial and intermediate cuneiforms, and base of the second metatarsal bone.[8] The ligamentous restraints serve to control transverse and sagittal motion.[12] Khaw and colleagues[13] confirmed the importance of these restraints by recognizing the effect of the plantar aponeurosis and first intermetatarsal ligament in stabilizing the TMT-1 and first ray. Although the first intermetatarsal ligament was shown to be a key stabilizer of the first metatarsal bone in all directions, the plantar aponeurosis was found to be an important secondary stabilizer resisting medial and dorsal rotation of the metatarsal after division of the first intermetatarsal ligament. Rush and colleagues[14] and Mizel[10] reported similar findings. The motion of the medial 3 TMT joints is minimal when compared with that of the 2 lateral ones. The center of rotation of the medial ray is found distal to the naviculocuneiform joint. As there is also a transversely directed force at the TMT-1, motion is not purely sagittal but rather 3-plane-like, running from dorsomedial to plantar-lateral, including eversion of the medial column because of the activation of the peroneus longus.[15,16] The peroneus longus and flexor hallucis longus muscles reduce dorsal instability.[17] Although the peroneus longus locks the medial cuneiform (first ray) into the medial column, through eversion of the first ray, it has no influence on transverse motion. In contrast, the flexor hallucis longus is able to possibly increase metatarsus primus varus deformity because of its pulling vector.[17] Increase of the 1–2 intermetatarsal angle results in loss of functional stability to the first ray provided by the plantar fascia.

HYPERMOBILITY OF THE FIRST RAY

Morton[1] was the first to introduce the concept of first ray hypermobility and its link to foot dysfunction in 1928. Later, Lapidus and Hansen believed that hypermobility of the first ray could be the cause of many forefoot derangements, for example, hallux valgus and central metatarsalgia.[3,18,19] Klaue and colleagues[20,21] were the first to propose hypermobility of the first ray as an important factor in the development of hallux valgus. However, no clear information exists to support this hypothesis. As stated by Rush and colleagues,[14] "a strict definition of first ray hypermobility remains elusive with its characterization being based predominantly on qualitative parameters." Hypermobility of the first ray cannot be precisely defined because proper identification of the abnormal motion at the TMT-1, the exact location of abnormal motion at the first ray, and its objective assessment are difficult. There is an innate difficulty of measuring the source of movements, which is additionally complicated by the choice of measurement methods. Movement occurs at the TMT-1, the naviculocuneiform, and talonavicular joints.[14,22,23] Assessment of motion at the TMT-1 joint has proved to be difficult. According to Ouzounian and Shereff[24] and Fritz and Prieskorn,[25] the motion at the TMT-1 joint averages 3.5° to 4.4° in flexion and extension and approximately 1.5° in pronation and supination (in contrast, motion at the fourth and fifth TMT joints averages 10° in flexion and extension and 10° in pronation and supination). Wanivenhaus and Pretterklieber[26] found no plantarflexion but 2.6° of dorsal extension. When trying to assess any hypermobility at the TMT-1 joint, it has been shown to be of value to measure either the dorsal or the plantar translation of the first metatarsal head and base. To accurately measure first ray mobility, Klaue and colleagues[21] described the use of a noninvasive caliper and defined a 1.5 ± 0.7-mm dorsal displacement of the first metatarsal base (5.3 ± 1.4-mm dorsal displacement of metatarsal head) in normal volunteers. In patients with hallux valgus, they found an average dorsal base displacement of 2.6 ± 1.4 mm and dorsal metatarsal head translation of 9.3 ± 1.9 mm. The device has recently been validated by Jones and colleagues[27] and found to be reliable. Similar to Klaue and colleagues, Glasoe and colleagues[22] used a mechanical device to measure first ray mobility and found a 4 mm dorsal displacement of the metatarsal head in the control group when compared with 6 mm in the subjects who had hallux valgus. Others attempted to quantify dorsal mobility by hypermobility of the TMT-1 using semimanual testing by means of small plastic plates (1 on the dorsal metatarsal and 1 on the dorsal second metatarsal).[28] They found that the first ray dorsal angular mobility was 10° in the normal group and 13° in the group that had hallux valgus.

First ray hypermobility in the sagittal plane is difficult to determine in the clinical setting. Hansen[19,29] described the manual testing of hypermobility at the first ray. Bednarz and Manoli[30] defined hypermobility manually to be as greater than 1 full thumb breadth of dorsal-to-plantar motion with the lesser toes stabilized. Voellmicke and Deland[31] performed manual testing by description of manual reference points and defined hypermobility as greater than 8 mm to 10 mm of dorsal displacement of the first metatarsal head when compared with the second metatarsal head. However, manual assessment is not reliable enough, and Glasoe and colleagues[22] questioned the validity of manual clinical testing because manual grading did not correlate with the absolute measurement of total dorsal mobility that was made by their device. A secondary radiographic finding, that is, the hypertrophy of the medial cortex of the second metatarsal (as an indirect sign of mechanical overload) has been discussed but not confirmed to be associated with first ray hypermobility.[16] Dorsal movement of the first ray in patients suffering from hallux valgus was found to be increased when compared with normal subjects. However, no clear correlation/association has been found between the amount of dorsal translation of the first ray and metatarsophalangeal and intermetatarsal angles.[28,32] Plantar gaping of the TMT-1 might indicate hypermobility.

THE EFFECT OF TMT-1 FUSION

From a logical standpoint, arthrodesis of the TMT-1 joint must have a biomechanical effect on the adjacent joints and/or function of the dynamic stabilizers, for example, the peroneus longus. In a biomechanical cadaveric study, Bierman and colleagues[33] showed that after fusion of the TMT-1, the regulatory function of the peroneus longus remained intact and eversion and plantarflexion of the first metatarsal was slightly greater than before fusion. Structural stability was increased while preserving the functional role of the peroneus longus in midstance phase. Additional fusion of the intercuneiform joint did not impair the function of the peroneus longus.

Fusion of the TMT-1 results in a longer lever arm and compensatory motion at the more proximally located joints, that is, the naviculocuneiform and talonavicular joints. As a result, the talus becomes dorsiflexed, heel to some extent inverted, and forefoot supinated.[33] Because of force transmissions into the proximal joints, degenerative changes could theoretically be induced. However, no data exist to reliably support and confirm this hypothesis.

PREOPERATIVE ASSESSMENT

The patient should be examined in the sitting, standing, and weight-bearing positions, which helps to demonstrate any magnitude of deformity and the effect of shoe wear on the foot. Inspection of the plantar aspect of the foot can reveal either localized or diffuse patterns of hyperkeratosis as a direct sign of load transmissions across the planta pedis. The toes are palpated and examined, and the range of motion is documented, along with plantarflexion and dorsiflexion of the ankle joint to accentuate and make visible contractures of the extensor or flexor tendons. Gastrocnemius or gastrocsoleus contracture is tested according to the method described by Silverskjöld. The neurovascular status should be carefully evaluated, with specific focus on the microcirculation of the lesser toes. This evaluation is important, as this circulation could be impaired in the postoperative phase, either because of improper handling of the soft tissues or preexisting capillary problems. Passive reduction of the TMT-1 is attempted. However, significant adduction contracture of the soft tissues could impair that maneuver. Manual testing of the first ray, albeit subjective, is used to assess hypermobility and done as described by Hansen. A dorsal translation of the metatarsal head of at least 1 shaft width could be considered as severe hypermobility of the first ray. Tenderness of the second metatarsophalangeal joint to palpation and pull could be a sign of synovitis caused by local overload.[16]

Standard weight-bearing foot radiographs, including anteroposterior, internal oblique, and lateral views, are sufficient to evaluate the forefoot. On the dorsoplantar view, the relative length of the first metatarsal in relation to the second should be evaluated and the congruity of the first metatarsophalangeal joint assessed. The 1–2 intermetatarsal angle (normal value ≤9°) is measured.[9] Medial hypertrophy of the second metatarsal cortex might be present but is not a reliable sign of first ray hypermobility. On the lateral view, the slopes of the metatarsals can be assessed and at times a plantar gaping of the TMT-1 is seen. More sophisticated diagnostic tools, such as computed tomography or magnetic resonance imaging, usually are not necessary.

GOALS AND INDICATIONS OF SURGERY

The primary goals of surgery are restoring alignment of the first metatarsal and improving its loading capacity, specifically in the presence of hypermobility. To achieve this, the correction is made at the apex of deformity. In general, hallux valgus deformities with metatarsophalangeal angles greater than 30° and 1–2 intermetatarsal angles of more than 18° provide indications for a TMT arthrodesis. TMT-1 fusions are also indicated to treat patients with hypermobility of the first ray, failed primary hallux valgus surgery, severe metatarsus primus elevatus, generalized ligamentous laxity, and arthritic changes of the TMT-1. Contraindications include a short first metatarsal; moderate hallux valgus deformities, which could be treated by distal metatarsal and/or phalangeal osteotomies; and open epiphyses in adolescents.[34,35] In case of a short first metatarsal, the interposition of a structural bone block should be considered.[19]

SURGICAL TECHNIQUE

Since its introduction many decades ago, the Lapidus procedure has seen several modifications and changes in technique and fixation. The goal of all those efforts was to improve primary stability at the fusion site and avoid excessive metatarsal shortening, which could lead to iatrogenic transfer metatarsalgia. Butson[36] and Giannestras[37] reported the use of the resected medial exostosis from the metatarsal head as bone graft in the TMT-1 to maintain the length of the first metatarsal relative to the second. Butson used temporary Kirschner wire (K wire) transfixation of the first metatarsal shaft to the second. Clark and colleagues[38] and, later, Sangeorzan and Hansen[39] introduced rigid screw fixation to obtain adequate compression and primary stability at the fusion site. In addition, in patients with a short first metatarsal, they incorporated a tricortical iliac crest autograft to restore length. To date, screw or plate fixation has become the preferred method of fixation. More recently, Saxena and colleagues[40] showed that the combination of a locking plate with a plantar screw allowed earlier weight bearing in comparison with crossed screws. Scranton and colleagues[41] evaluated the strength of locking plates and found it to be superior when compared with crossed screws alone. Klos and colleagues[42] reported similar results. In conclusion, the combination of a medial locking plate with a plantar compression screw shows promising results and could help to reduce the weight-bearing period and rate of nonunions.

Modified Lapidus Procedure

1. Exposure and preparation of the TMT-1 (**Figs. 1** and **2**)
    A dorsomedial incision next to the extensor hallucis longus tendon (anatomic landmark) is made
    Care is taken not to injure the sensory branch of the superficial peroneal nerve and the dorsalis pedis artery
    The capsule is exposed and incised
    The articular surfaces are debrided from their cartilage with an osteotome

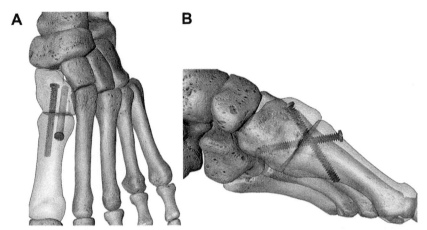

Fig. 1. (*A, B*) Three-dimensional renderings including the dorsoplantar and lateral views of the foot. Depicted is the technique of the modified Lapidus procedure using 2 crossing and compressing screws.

A small oscillating saw is used to trim the lateral aspect of the base of the first metatarsal, the lateral aspect of the medial cuneiform (allows better lateral translation and rotation of the first metatarsal), and the plantar ridge of the medial cuneiform (avoids extension malunion)

The articular surfaces are drilled with a 1.5-mm drill bit to prepare them for fusion

The first metatarsal is pushed laterally and slightly plantarly and temporarily fixed with a K wire

The first 3.5-mm screw is inserted from distal into the plantar medial aspect of the medial cuneiform

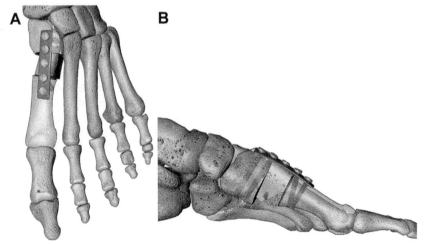

Fig. 2. (*A, B*) This 3-dimensional image illustrates how a tricortical iliac crest graft is inserted between the metatarsal shaft and medial cuneiform and secured by means of screws and plates. Additional reinforcement can be achieved by inserting an oblique screw directed from the base of the first metatarsal to the intermediate cuneiform.

    The second 3.5-mm screw is inserted from the medial cuneiform to the plantar base of the first metatarsal

    Sometimes a third 3.5-mm screw is needed to obtain more stability or in case of excessive hypermobility

    If there is marked shortening of the first ray, an autologous iliac crest graft can be inserted. In such a case, plate fixation might be necessary to achieve better stability and ensure union (see **Fig. 2**).

2. Exposure and preparation of the first metatarsophalangeal joint

    A medial incision over the first metatarsophalangeal joint is made

    The neurovascular bundle is exposed dorsomedially and carefully retracted to lateral

    A longitudinal incision of the capsule is made

    The lateral capsule is reached from medial and transversely incised (the adductor tendon should not be detached)

    In case of insufficient correction, an Akin osteotomy or even chevron osteotomy could be considered.

3. Postoperative care

    The patient's foot is placed in a plaster-of-Paris cast

    Two days postoperatively the cast is removed, and the foot is placed in a Soft Cast (3M, St Paul, MN, USA)

    The patient is kept non–weight bearing with 2 crutches for 8 weeks

    If fusion is complete, the patient receives physical therapy and progressive weight-bearing status.

OUTCOME

The literature reveals reliable and adequate correction of moderate to severe grades of metatarsus primus varus and hallux valgus and patient satisfaction rates from 74% to 96%.[30,39] As reported by many investigators, there is successful pain relief from symptomatic hallux valgus. Modifications of the procedure and improved preparation and fixation methods result in low incidences of recurrence and nonunion (**Figs. 3–5**). However, only few prospective studies on Lapidus procedures are available. Listing all scientific articles on this topic is beyond the scope of the present review; only the most important articles are discussed here. The Seattle group was one of the first to report on the modified Lapidus procedure for the treatment of symptomatic hallux valgus with hypermobile first ray.[38,39] The retrospective results in 32 patients (40 feet) who were operated on were evaluated. Preoperative diagnosis was symptomatic hallux valgus with a hypermobile first ray in 33 feet and failed bunion surgery in 7. The minimal follow-up period was 30 months. Ninety percent of fusions achieved complete union. The 1–2 intermetatarsal angle was corrected from 14° preoperatively to 6° postoperatively. The average change in the length of the first metatarsal was −5 mm for those without a bone graft and +4 mm for those with a bone graft (**Fig. 6**). Seventy-five percent of cases were judged as successfully corrected. All the 7 feet operated on for failed previous surgery improved. The investigators found the best results obtained in those patients who had a multiple screw fixation, use of bone graft, and attention to plantarflexion of the first metatarsal. Myerson and coworkers[34] presented their results of the Lapidus procedure in 53 patients (67 feet). The metatarsophalangeal angle was corrected by 20° and the intermetatarsal angle by approximately 10°. Range of motion at the first metatarsophalangeal joint after the procedure was 85% of normal. About 77% of patients were completely relieved, 15% partially relieved, and 8% not relieved with respect to pain, comfort, foot appearance, and

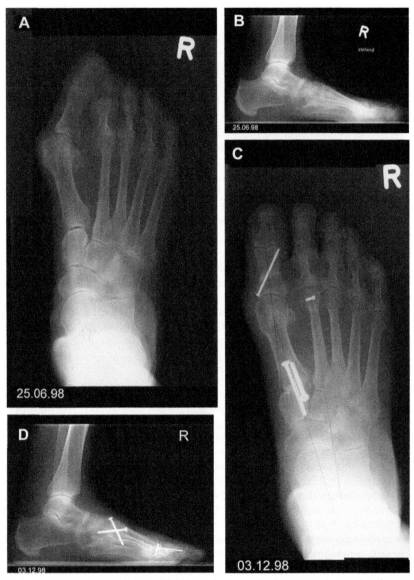

Fig. 3. Preoperative dorsoplantar (*A*) and lateral (*B*) weight-bearing radiographs of a patient with hallux valgus deformity associated with hypermobility of the first ray. On the lateral radiograph, a slight plantar gaping of the TMT-1 can be noticed. (*C, D*) Postoperative dorsoplantar and lateral radiographs of the same patient as in **Fig. 3**A, B. The patient was treated by a modified Lapidus procedure combined with an Akin osteotomy to correct the hallux valgus deformity distally. To prevent transfer metatarsalgia, a Weil osteotomy was added on the second metatarsal.

shoe wear. Others investigated the intermediate outcome in 26 patients (31 feet) who underwent a modified Lapidus procedure for the treatment of hallux valgus secondary to a hypermobile first ray.[30] All patients but one (96%) were satisfied with the surgery. Postoperative pain relief was totally satisfying in 73% and satisfying with reservations

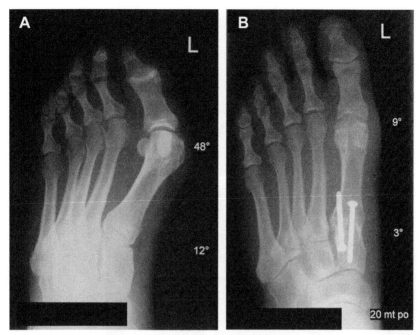

Fig. 4. (*A*) Dorsoplantar weight-bearing radiograph of a patient with hypermobility of the first ray. The first metatarsophalangeal angle measures 48°, and the intermetatarsal angle, 12°. (*B*) To correct the hallux valgus deformity and treat hypermobility, the patient was treated by the modified 2-screws Lapidus technique.

in 23% of patients. One patient (4%) was not satisfied. No stiffness at the first metatarsophalangeal joint was found in 22 patients, noticeable but not bothersome stiffness in 3 patients, and stiffness that impairs activity in 1 patient (2 feet). The average improvement of the metatarsophalangeal angle and the intermetatarsal angle was 10°. Coetzee and Wickum[43] in a prospective outcome study of 91 patients (105 feet; average age, 41 years) reported a significant improvement of the American Orthopaedic Foot and Ankle Society (AOFAS) scores after a mean follow-up of 4 years. All patients had moderate to severe hallux valgus deformities and were treated with a Lapidus procedure. The studies of Bednarz and Manoli[30] and Myerson and colleagues[34] showed that the metatarsophalangeal and 1–2 intermetatarsal angles could successfully be corrected by approximately 20° and 10°, respectively. Metatarsophalangeal and 1–2 intermetatarsal angles did not significantly increase between the first and last year of follow-up.

Thompson and colleagues[44] performed a large retrospective study of 182 patients and recommended meticulous preparation of the joint and the use of a graft with local autologous bone to achieve good clinical and radiologic outcomes. The investigators found that patients with previous bunion surgery and recurrent deformity were at a higher risk for a nonunion.

More recently, Kopp and colleagues[45] confirmed the power of correction of the modified Lapidus procedure with almost the exactly same amount of hallux valgus and intermetatarsal angle correction when compared with the previously mentioned studies. Ninety percent of patients were satisfied with foot function.

A retrospective study of prospectively collected cohort data evaluated the functional outcomes and patient satisfaction after Lapidus procedures for the treatment

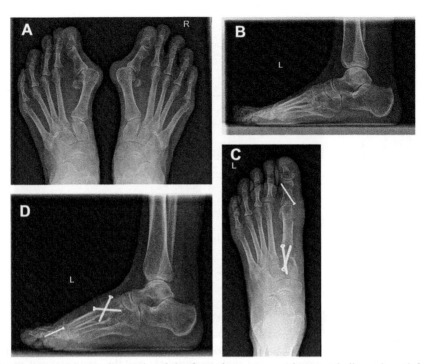

Fig. 5. Conventional radiographs of the feet of a woman with severe hallux valgus deformity associated with metatarsus primus varus and hypermobility of the first ray (dorsoplantar [A] and lateral [B] views). Note the large intermetatarsal angle. (C, D) Postoperative dorsoplantar (C) and lateral (D) views of the left foot of the same patient as mentioned in **Fig. 5**A, B. Note the correction of the intermetatarsal angle. An Akin procedure was performed with a lateral soft tissue release of the first metatarsophalangeal joint.

of failed hallux valgus surgery.[46,47] For this purpose, 24 patients (26 feet) were reviewed after 24 months. The final AOFAS score averaged 88 points, and the metatarsophalangeal angle improved by 20°. Similar to the results obtained by primary fusion of the first metatarsocuneiform joint, the 1–2 intermetatarsal angle was decreased by approximately 10°. No patient was dissatisfied at the time of the follow-up. No hallux varus occurred in the study group. The investigators concluded that the Lapidus procedure was a reliable and effective treatment of recurrent hallux valgus deformity.

COMPLICATIONS

The most important complications of a Lapidus procedure include nonunion, malunion, recurrence of primary deformity, and transfer metatarsalgia. Nonunion rates have been reported to range between 0% and 16%.[34,36,38,39,48–52] Malunion, that is, dorsal elevation of the first metatarsal, may occur in up to 9%.[34] Revision rates due to pain, however, range between 2% and 13%.[39,51,53] Nonunions seem to occur predominantly in smokers.[43] A recent study showed that the reoperation rate for hallux valgus averaged 2.92% and that for hallux varus averaged 0.29%.[53] Recurrence of deformity has been found to range from 0% to 16%.[30,34,39,43,45,48,51,53–55]

Hallux varus is a serious complication and might occur long after the initial procedures. Rates between 8% and 16% were reported in the literature.[45,49] However,

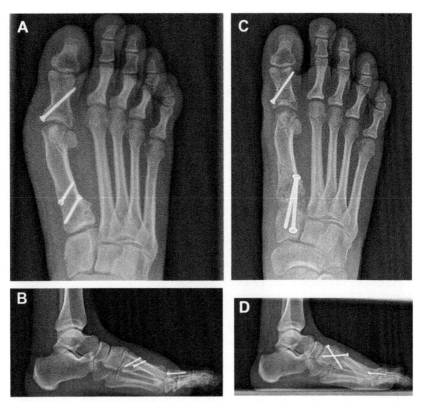

Fig. 6. (*A, B*) Preoperative radiographs of a young female patient who has been treated several times for symptomatic hallux valgus deformity. The clinical examination revealed a recurrent hallux valgus deformity and transfer metatarsalgia as a result of the short first metatarsal and gross instability of the first ray. Based on those findings, a Lapidus procedure combined with interposition of a tricortical iliac crest graft was performed. Dorsoplantar (*C*) and lateral (*D*) views of the foot 8 weeks after modified Lapidus procedure combined with interposition of an iliac crest autograft. Note the callus formation dorsal to the first meta-tarsocuneiform *joint*.

most of those cases are attributable to the distal soft tissue release performed to realign the first metatarsophalangeal joint rather than to the TMT-1 arthrodesis. The rate of transfer metatarsalgia ranges from 4% to 5%,[43,56] which is because of the excessive shortening of the first metatarsal and possible dorsal malunion of the first metatarsal.[57]

Subjective complaint of foot stiffness has been reported to range between 8% and 18%.[34,35,58] Other complications include deep vein thrombosis, wound infections, and nerve lesions.

SUMMARY

The modified Lapidus procedure represents a powerful tool to correct various forefoot abnormalities, including conditions after failed bunion surgery and hallux valgus deformity associated with hypermobility of the first ray. Because of the advanced knowledge of fusion techniques and fixation methods, the procedure provides good to excellent patient satisfaction in most individuals and adequate correction of metatarsophalangeal and intermetatarsal angles.

REFERENCES

1. Morton D, editor. The human foot. New York: Columbia University Press; 1935.
2. Courriades H. L'hypermobilite du premier rayon. Podologie 1971;6:146–53 [in French].
3. Lapidus PW. A quarter of a century of experience with the operative correction of the metatarsus varus primus in hallux valgus. Bull Hosp Joint Dis 1956;17(2):404–21.
4. Truslow W. Metatarsus primus varus or hallux valgus? J Bone Joint Surg Am 1925; 7:98.
5. Kleinberg S. Operative cure of hallux valgus and bunions. Am J Surg 1932;15:75–81.
6. Ridola CG, Cappello F, Marciano V, et al. The synovial joints of the human foot. Ital J Anat Embryol 2007;112(2):61–80.
7. Lapidus PW. Kinesiology and mechanical anatomy of the tarsal joints. Clin Orthop Relat Res 1963;30:20–36.
8. Sarrafian SK, editor. Anatomy of the foot and ankle: descriptive, topographic, functional. Philadelphia: JB Lippincott; 1983.
9. Hardy R, Clapham J. Observations on hallux valgus. J Bone Joint Surg Br 1951; 33(3):376–91.
10. Mizel MS. The role of the plantar first metatarsal first cuneiform ligament in weightbearing on the first metatarsal. Foot Ankle 1993;14(2):82–4.
11. Solan MC, Moorman CT 3rd, Miyamoto RG, et al. Ligamentous restraints of the second tarsometatarsal joint: a biomechanical evaluation. Foot Ankle Int 2001; 22(8):637–41.
12. Kuhlmann JN, Guerin-Surville H, Baux S. [The intermetatarsal transverse ligaments and their connections with the tarsometatarsal articulations]. Bull Assoc Anat (Nancy) 1992;76(234):19–27 [in French].
13. Khaw FM, Mak P, Johnson GR, et al. Distal ligamentous restraints of the first metatarsal. An in vitro biomechanical study. Clin Biomech (Bristol, Avon) 2005;20(6): 653–8.
14. Rush SM, Christensen JC, Johnson CH. Biomechanics of the first ray. Part II: metatarsus primus varus as a cause of hypermobility. A three-dimensional kinematic analysis in a cadaver model. J Foot Ankle Surg 2000;39(2):68–77.
15. Faber FW, Kleinrensink GJ, Verhoog MW, et al. Mobility of the first tarsometatarsal joint in relation to hallux valgus deformity: anatomical and biomechanical aspects. Foot Ankle Int 1999;20(10):651–6.
16. Faber FW, Kleinrensink GJ, Mulder PG, et al. Mobility of the first tarsometatarsal joint in hallux valgus patients: a radiographic analysis. Foot Ankle Int 2001;22(12): 965–9.
17. Johnson CH, Christensen JC. Biomechanics of the first ray. Part I. The effects of peroneus longus function: a three-dimensional kinematic study on a cadaver model. J Foot Ankle Surg 1999;38(5):313–21.
18. Maguire W. The Lapidus procedure for hallux valgus. J Bone Joint Surg Br 1973; 55:221.
19. Hansen ST, editor. Functional reconstruction of the foot and ankle. Philadelphia: Lippincott Williams and Wilkins; 2000. p. 145–86.
20. Klaue K. [Hallux valgus and hypermobility of the first ray–causal treatment using tarso-metatarsal reorientation arthrodesis]. Ther Umsch 1991;48(12):817–23 [in German].

21. Klaue K, Hansen ST, Masquelet AC. Clinical, quantitative assessment of first tarsometatarsal mobility in the sagittal plane and its relation to hallux valgus deformity. Foot Ankle Int 1994;15(1):9–13.
22. Glasoe WM, Yack HJ, Saltzman CL. Measuring first ray mobility with a new device. Arch Phys Med Rehabil 1999;80(1):122–4.
23. Myerson MS, Badekas A. Hypermobility of the first ray. Foot Ankle Clin 2000;5(3):469–84.
24. Ouzounian TJ, Shereff MJ. Common ankle disorders of the elderly: diagnosis and management. Geriatrics 1988;43(12):73–80.
25. Fritz GR, Prieskorn D. First metatarsocuneiform motion: a radiographic and statistical analysis. Foot Ankle Int 1995;16(3):117–23.
26. Wanivenhaus A, Pretterklieber M. First tarsometatarsal joint: anatomical biomechanical study. Foot Ankle 1989;9(4):153–7.
27. Jones CP, Coughlin MJ, Pierce-Villadot R, et al. The validity and reliability of the Klaue device. Foot Ankle Int 2005;26(11):951–6.
28. Lee KT, Young K. Measurement of first-ray mobility in normal vs. hallux valgus patients. Foot Ankle Int 2001;22(12):960–4.
29. Hansen ST Jr. Hallux valgus surgery. Morton and Lapidus were right! Clin Podiatr Med Surg 1996;13(3):347–54.
30. Bednarz PA, Manoli A 2nd. Modified lapidus procedure for the treatment of hypermobile hallux valgus. Foot Ankle Int 2000;21(10):816–21.
31. Voellmicke KV, Deland JT. Manual examination technique to assess dorsal instability of the first ray. Foot Ankle Int 2002;23(11):1040–1.
32. Glasoe WM, Allen MK, Ludewig PM. Comparison of first ray dorsal mobility among different forefoot alignments. J Orthop Sports Phys Ther 2000;30(10):612–20 [discussion: 621–3].
33. Bierman RA, Christensen JC, Johnson CH. Biomechanics of the first ray. Part III. Consequences of Lapidus arthrodesis on peroneus longus function: a three-dimensional kinematic analysis in a cadaver model. J Foot Ankle Surg 2001;40(3):125–31.
34. Myerson M, Allon S, McGarvey W. Metatarsocuneiform arthrodesis for management of hallux valgus and metatarsus primus varus. Foot Ankle 1992;13(3):107–15.
35. Myerson M. Metatarsocuneiform arthrodesis for treatment of hallux valgus and metatarsus primus varus. Orthopedics 1990;13(9):1025–31.
36. Butson AR. A modification of the Lapidus operation for hallux valgus. J Bone Joint Surg Br 1980;62(3):350–2.
37. Giannestras N. The Giannestras modification of the Lapidus operation. In: Giannestras N, editor. Foot disorders: medical and surgical management. Philadelphia: Lea & Febiger; 1973.
38. Clark HR, Veith RG, Hansen ST Jr. Adolescent bunions treated by the modified Lapidus procedure. Bull Hosp Jt Dis Orthop Inst 1987;47(2):109–22.
39. Sangeorzan BJ, Hansen ST Jr. Modified Lapidus procedure for hallux valgus. Foot Ankle 1989;9(6):262–6.
40. Saxena A, Nguyen A, Nelsen E. Lapidus bunionectomy: Early evaluation of crossed lag screws versus locking plate with plantar lag screw. J Foot Ankle Surg 2009;48(2):170–9.
41. Scranton PE, Coetzee JC, Carreira D. Arthrodesis of the first metatarsocuneiform joint: a comparative study of fixation methods. Foot Ankle Int 2009;30(4):341–5.
42. Klos K, Gueorguiev B, Muckley T, et al. Stability of medial locking plate and compression screw versus two crossed screws for Lapidus arthrodesis. Foot Ankle Int 2010;31(2):158–63.

43. Coetzee JC, Wickum D. The Lapidus procedure: a prospective cohort outcome study. Foot Ankle Int 2004;25(8):526–31.

44. Thompson IM, Bohay DR, Anderson JG. Fusion rate of first tarsometatarsal arthrodesis in the modified Lapidus procedure and flatfoot reconstruction. Foot Ankle Int 2005;26(9):698–703.

45. Kopp FJ, Patel MM, Levine DS, et al. The modified Lapidus procedure for hallux valgus: a clinical and radiographic analysis. Foot Ankle Int 2005;26(11):913–7.

46. Coetzee JC, Resig SG, Kuskowski M, et al. The Lapidus procedure as salvage after failed surgical treatment of hallux valgus: a prospective cohort study. J Bone Joint Surg Am 2003;85(1):60–5.

47. Coetzee JC, Resig SG, Kuskowski M, et al. The Lapidus procedure as salvage after failed surgical treatment of hallux valgus. Surgical technique. J Bone Joint Surg Am 2004;86(Suppl 1):30–6.

48. Patel S, Ford LA, Etcheverry J, et al. Modified lapidus arthrodesis: rate of nonunion in 227 cases. J Foot Ankle Surg 2004;43(1):37–42.

49. Mauldin DM, Sanders M, Whitmer WW. Correction of hallux valgus with metatarsocuneiform stabilization. Foot Ankle 1990;11(2):59–66.

50. Catanzariti AR, Mendicino RW, Lee MS, et al. The modified Lapidus arthrodesis: a retrospective analysis. J Foot Ankle Surg 1999;38(5):322–32.

51. McInnes BD, Bouche RT. Critical evaluation of the modified Lapidus procedure. J Foot Ankle Surg 2001;40(2):71–90.

52. Grace D, Delmonte R, Catanzariti AR, et al. Modified lapidus arthrodesis for adolescent hallux abducto valgus. J Foot Ankle Surg 1999;38(1):8–13.

53. Lagaay PM, Hamilton GA, Ford LA, et al. Rates of revision surgery using Chevron-Austin osteotomy, Lapidus arthrodesis, and closing base wedge osteotomy for correction of hallux valgus deformity. J Foot Ankle Surg 2008;47(4):267–72.

54. Treadwell JR. Rail external fixation for stabilization of closing base wedge osteotomies and Lapidus procedures: a retrospective analysis of sixteen cases. J Foot Ankle Surg 2005;44(6):429–36.

55. Fuhrmann RA. Arthrodesis of the first tarsometatarsal joint for correction of the advanced splayfoot accompanied by a hallux valgus. Oper Orthop Traumatol 2005;17(2):195–210.

56. Rink-Brune O. Lapidus arthrodesis for management of hallux valgus–a retrospective review of 106 cases. J Foot Ankle Surg 2004;43(5):290–5.

57. Espinosa N, Brodsky JW, Maceira E. Metatarsalgia. J Am Acad Orthop Surg 2010;18(8):474–85.

58. Schon LC, Myerson MS. Cuneiform-metatarsal arthrodesis for hallux valgus. In: Kitaoka HB, editor. The foot and ankle. Philadelphia: Lippincott Williams & Wilkins; 2002. p. 99–117.

Surgical Correction of Midfoot Arthritis With and Without Deformity

Alan J. Zonno, MD, Mark S. Myerson, MD*

KEYWORDS

• Midfoot arthritis • Surgical correction • Deformity • Arthrodesis

The goals of any midfoot reconstruction are to create a painless, functional, and plantigrade foot, which is generally accomplished with arthrodesis and which must be performed with realignment. The latter requires not only the correction of any midfoot deformity when present but also coexisting forefoot and hindfoot deformities. The more significant of these deformities is in the hindfoot, because heel valgus leads to persistent problems and even recurrent deformity of the midfoot.

PATTERNS OF DEFORMITY

Posttraumatic deformities are a common cause of midfoot arthritis, although with changing demographics of an older population, primary osteoarthritis is the more common cause of deformity. Inflammatory disorders and diabetic neuroarthropathy are also commonly implicated in the development of midfoot arthrosis and collapse of the medial longitudinal arch. Less commonly discussed causes of midfoot arthritis include first ray instability, brachymetatarsia of the first metatarsal (MT), and a long second MT.[1] Regardless of presumed cause, careful physical examination and review of radiographic studies are essential to detect and treat patterns of midfoot deformity.

Increased stress placed on the longitudinal arch with weight bearing after midfoot ligamentous disruption results in variable collapse of the longitudinal arch and subsequent disruption of force transmission from the hindfoot to the forefoot. After Lisfranc injury, Schepers and colleagues[2] reported reduced contact time of the forefoot as well as increased contacted surface area and higher maximum pressures at the midfoot. Compensatory gait patterns and pain (in the absence of neuropathy) ensue. Dorsal

Disclosure: Dr Myerson is a consultant to Orthohelix, Extremity Medical, and DePuy.
The Institute for Foot and Ankle Reconstruction, Mercy Medical Center, 301 St Paul Place, Baltimore, MD 21202, USA
* Corresponding author.
E-mail address: mark4feet@aol.com

osteophytes cause difficulty with shoe wear, whereas plantar osteophytes result in callus formation and ulceration. Common deformities associated with tarsometatarsal (TMT) joint arthritis and longitudinal arch collapse include forefoot abduction, sagittal and coronal abnormalities of the midfoot, and hindfoot valgus. Jung and colleagues[3] further describe 4 main operative subtypes observed with atraumatic TMT degenerative joint disease, including pes planovalgus, hallux valgus, in situ without deformity, and rocker bottom deformity.

SURGICAL DECISION MAKING

The heterogeneity of deformities encountered makes treatment protocols difficult to formulate and adhere to on a regular basis. However, the most important issue is which joints to fuse and whether or not realignment is necessary. Sangeorzan and colleagues[4] reported that the only useful factor to determine outcome after fixation of TMT joint injuries was alignment. In situ fusion is indicated only in cases of slight deformity (<2 mm displacement and <15° angulation).[5] Deformity exceeding these parameters is an indication for realignment during arthrodesis.

Realignment begins at the apex of the deformity, which is generally located at the medial column of the TMT joint complex. Rarely, if there is a severe adduction deformity associated with collapse and erosion of the first metatarsocuneiform joint, the apex of the deformity is laterally based at the fifth MT, which is therefore realigned first. The talus-first MT axis needs to be reestablished in both the sagittal and transverse planes. The medial base of the first MT should be in line with the medial wall of the medial cuneiform, and the medial base of the second MT should be in line with the medial edge of the middle cuneiform. If lateral column realignment and fusion are required, the medial base of the 4th MT should be in line with the medial edge of the cuboid.

Correction of concurrent hindfoot deformities can be accomplished according to the sequence outlined by Den Hartog and Kay,[6] which requires sequential realignment from proximal to distal in the following manner: (1) gastrocnemius soleus complex contracture; (2) hindfoot malalignment; (3) forefoot supination-pronation; (4) forefoot abduction-adduction; (5) rocker bottom deformity; and (6) multiplanar deformity. Gastrocnemius or Achilles contracture is addressed with either a gastrocnemius recession or percutaneous Achilles lengthening, respectively. If the hindfoot is left in equinus there is too much force on the midfoot, and recurrent deformity, particularly associated with medial column instability, can develop. Hindfoot valgus is corrected with a medial translational calcaneal osteotomy (varus deformity does not typically occur in conjunction with midfoot arthritis). If the heel is left in valgus, there is increased pronation and abduction on the midfoot, and further deformity may develop. For example, if a TMT arthrodesis has been performed, arthritis can develop at the naviculocuneiform joint. The realignment of the midfoot and forefoot must include pronation-supination and abduction-adduction malalignment, and is corrected using rotation and angulation after adequate debridement and joint preparation. We are not likely to use resection of wedges to correct deformity. Although biplanar wedge resection of the TMT joints can correct deformity in both the sagittal and transverse planes, it severely shortens the foot. However, in the neuropathic foot, this procedure may be necessary.

So how best to decide which joints to include in the arthrodesis? Those that are symptomatic should be included, but this is not always easy to define, particularly because the lateral column is often asymptomatic despite radiographic evidence of arthrosis. A paradox exists in that the least mobile joints within the TMT complex (the middle column) are the ones that are the most frequently involved in painful arthritis. The lateral column is the most mobile in both dorsiflexion-plantarflexion and pronation-supination.[7] However, maintenance of lateral column motion is important for optimal function after midfoot arthrodesis.[5] Therefore it is not surprising that routine inclusion of the lateral column in midfoot fusion has not been recommended.[4,5] Although Raikin and Schon[8] reported improvements in function after lateral column arthrodesis, most patients in this study had neuropathy, and the indication for lateral column inclusion in the fusion construct included uncorrectable lateral midfoot collapse with rocker bottom deformity. **Fig. 1** shows TMT joint arthrodesis involving all 3 columns. An alternative to fusing all 3 columns of the TMT joint complex is arthrodesis of the medial and middle columns, supplemented by interposition arthroplasty or cheilectomy (which is our preference) of the lateral column.

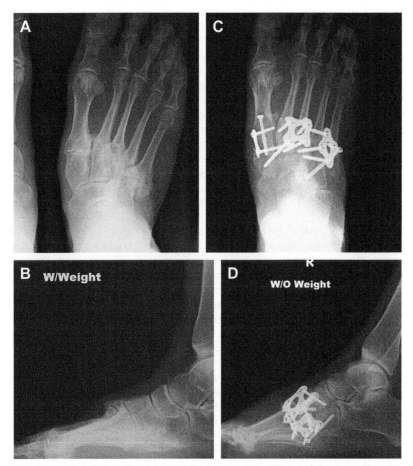

Fig. 1. Three-column fusion. (*A, B*) This patient presented with painful primary degenerative arthritis involving all 5 TMT joints. (*C, D*) Realignment and fusion of all 3 columns was performed. However, our current recommended treatment of symptomatic lateral column arthrosis without neuropathic collapse is cheilectomy at the fourth and fifth MT-cuboid articulations to preserve motion.

Once the initial decisions have been made regarding realignment and which joints to include in the arthrodesis, the surgical plan should take into account the following elements: surgical approach, arthrodesis preparation, order of fixation, and choice of fixation construct. In addition, special attention should be given to soft tissue considerations and the use of bone graft and osteobiologic agents.

SURGICAL APPROACHES

Multiple longitudinal incisions are generally accepted, because the number of parallel incisions can be modified according to the planned arthrodesis. If only the first and second TMT joints are to be fused, a single dorsal incision in the first-second MT interspace can be used if minimal deformity is present. A 2-incision approach is recommended in the presence of more severe deformity, medial column instability, or for the removal of plantar osteophytes. If the medial and middle columns are included, then either 1 or 2 incisions are used, again depending on the presence of medial column instability and plantar osteophytes. These osteophytes are the result of instability of the first TMT joint and cause painful buildup of callosity under the plantar medial foot. They must be removed, and therefore the medial column is approached from a medial midline incision that facilitates access to the first TMT joint as well as the naviculocuneiform joint as needed. The anterior tibial tendon attaches over the surface of the medial cuneiform and cannot be protected. We prefer to cut directly through the tendon insertion if it blocks exposure, and then to repair the tendon after screw of plate fixation. The second and third TMT joints are accessed through a second parallel incision centered between the second and third MTs. Be careful with the latter incision, because one has a tendency to err too far medially over the second MT, making exposure of the third TMT joint difficult. A third parallel incision between the fourth and fifth MTs can be used if access to the lateral column is desirable. Alternatively, an isolated middle column fusion can be approached with a single longitudinal incision just lateral to the second MT.

The 3-incision approach[5] for the correction of severe deformity is useful, although Vertullo and colleagues[9] reported the use of a single transverse dorsal incision to expose the midfoot. Complications we have encountered with longitudinal dorsal incisions include bruising, dehiscence, and necrosis of the margins of the incision, which generally are the result of overretraction. This situation makes a transverse dorsal incision more appealing, because it should theoretically minimize the risk of wound necrosis associated with inadequate skin bridges and the disruption of subcutaneous blood supply.[9] We have used this transverse incision successfully in patients with neuropathy when the concern for transection of a branch of the superficial peroneal or deep peroneal nerve is not so significant. This transverse incision is centered over the TMT joints and can be extended into a medially based T-incision for extended medial column access. Regardless of the incisions used, full thickness flaps are raised to minimize the risk of devascularization of the subcutaneous tissues, and branches of the superficial peroneal nerve must be protected. The tendon of the extensor hallucis brevis should be located and used as a guide to identify the deep neurovascular bundle, which lies just inferior to it. Generally we retract the tendon, but if necessary, it can be cut to improve exposure. One has to be careful with the use of this transverse dorsal incision if the midfoot or TMT joints are dorsally and proximally dislocated. When reducing the joints there is increased tension on the skin, leading to dehiscence. Therefore with a complete dislocation we are more likely to use longitudinal incisions.

ARTHRODESIS PREPARATION

Although realignment is important, the key to this procedure is the correct and adequate debridement and preparation of the joint spaces. A combination of chisels and curettes followed by perforation of the subchondral bone with a 2-mm drill to create a slurry of bone in the joint space is ideal. It is preferable to retain the overall architecture of each TMT joint. When the fusion involves the first and second TMT joints, the interspace between the bases of the MTs can also be prepared and included in the arthrodesis (**Fig. 2**). It is important to adequately debride the plantar surface of each TMT joint, and a smooth laminar spreader is particularly helpful to provide distraction during the preparation of the deeper plantar joint space. If this is not done, plantar joint debris is left behind, which results in dorsiflexion of the arthrodesis, a dorsal malunion, and metatarsalgia. If a dorsal malunion of the first TMT joint occurs, it also restricts dorsiflexion of the hallux metatarsophalangeal joint. If adjacent TMT joints are fused, their respective intercuneiform joint spaces can also be debrided and fused.

Bone graft and osteobiologic agents are generally not required for primary arthrodesis. Nevertheless, local autologous bone graft obtained from the drill used to prepare the joint spaces can be packed into the TMT and intercuneiform joint spaces (see **Fig. 2**). Structural bone graft, on the other hand, may be required for deformity realignment. The primary sources of structural bone graft are either autologous iliac crest harvested at the time of surgery or structural allograft with or without the addition of autologous stem cells that we typically harvest from the concentrate of the iliac crest aspirate. Although published data are scarce regarding the use of structural allograft for midfoot deformity correction, Myerson and colleagues[10] reported on 3 cases of

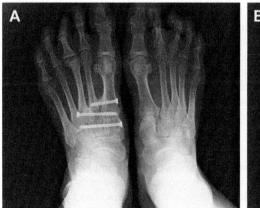
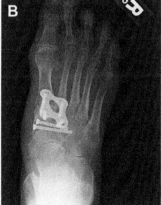

Fig. 2. Arthrodesis involving the medial and middle columns. (*A*) In addition to the incongruity between the medial aspect of the second MT and the medial aspect of the middle cuneiform, note the instability that exists between the medial and middle cuneiforms. The planned fusion construct included the first and second TMT articulations as well as the intercuneiform space. (*B*) After screw fixation across the intercuneiform space, a 4-hole Maxlock Extreme plate (OrthoHelix, Medina, OH, USA) was chosen. Its precontoured design permits fixation of all 4 bones in the fusion construct. The plate provides axial as well as coronal stability, and allows compression across the first and second TMT articulations. A central hole in the plate permits the use of local bone graft in the interspace between the bases of the first and second MTs.

TMT structural allograft in a study of 75 patients for whom structural allograft was used. It is important to restore the length and alignment, particularly of the medial column, and for these cases it is not adequate to use cancellous graft. The insertion of structural graft can be difficult, and it is necessary to distract the medial column before inserting the graft. This procedure can be carried out with a smooth laminar spreader (**Fig. 3**C) or a pin distractor, wedging the graft into place under compression. **Figs. 3** and **4** show the use of structural allograft for realignment with midfoot fusion.

ORDER OF FIXATION

The medial column is generally stabilized first to create stability for the remainder of the midfoot. The reduction of the medial column is accomplished by 3 simultaneous maneuvers: hallux dorsiflexion forces the first MT into plantarflexion and simultaneously compresses the joint. Be careful not to overplantarflex the first MT because sesamoiditis occurs, which can be refractory to treatment because of the rigidity of the MT. With the hallux dorsiflexed, axial pressure along the first MT increases impaction of the MT base into the medial cuneiform. The first MT must be slightly adducted so that its base is colinear with the medial cuneiform. The latter can be difficult to assess, particularly if there is an abduction deformity to begin with, and it may be useful to compare the alignment with the contralateral radiograph to verify correction.

Provisional fixation is accomplished with K-wires or cannulated screw guide wires, but these should be inserted axially because an oblique wire or guide pin interferes with compression across the joint. The second MT is subsequently reduced into its mortise and held with a bone reduction clamp between the lateral base of the second MT and the proximal aspect of the medial cuneiform. It is helpful to insert a guide pin for cannulated screw fixation along the plane of reduction, sometimes referred to as a Lisfranc screw. This technique does not provide any compression for arthrodesis, but does maintain reduction and improve alignment. Regardless of the technique used, intercuneiform instability must be recognized and managed before the reduction of the second TMT joint. If there is significant widening between the medial and middle cuneiforms, then a second reduction clamp should be used, applying compression across the midfoot. Sequential fusion of the third TMT joint is indicated if it is symptomatic, unstable, or part of the deformity correction. Arthrodesis of the lateral column is not performed routinely. However, it may be indicated as part of a neuropathic, degenerative, or posttraumatic process with a lateral rocker bottom deformity.

CHOICE OF FIXATION

The goal of fixation is stability that allows sufficient time for complete arthrodesis. The ideal fixation is one that provides stability, compression, and is versatile enough to include 1 or more of the midfoot joints. Screws can be used, and should be large enough to provide sufficient stability, such as a 3.5-mm fully threaded screw introduced with a lag technique or a 4.0-mm partially threaded screw. The key to screw fixation is to avoid splitting the base of the MT with the final few turns of the screwdriver. This situation is unpredictable and even with a good countersink technique still occurs. We prefer not to use the countersink provided in the screw set, but to use a burr to create a well for the head of the screw. It is straightforward to insert 2 axial screws across the first metatarsocuneiform joint, one from proximal and lateral aimed distal and plantar, and the second from dorsal distal and medial aimed proximally and medially. However, this procedure is not so easy with the second and third MTs, and for this reason we use a custom plate for the midfoot (**Fig. 5**), which provides good

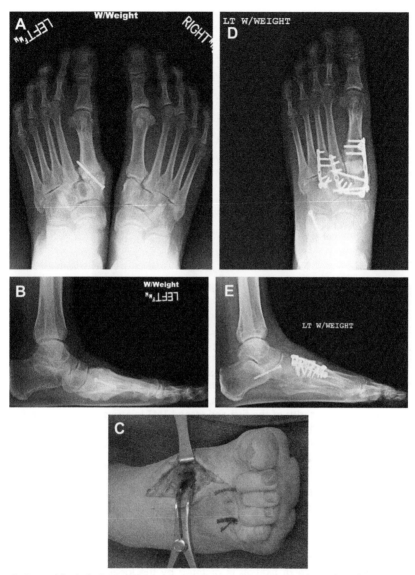

Fig. 3. Bone block fusion with symptomatic transfer metatarsalgia. (*A, B*) Preoperative radiographs reveal arthrosis of the medial and middle columns after malreduction of a Lisfranc injury with midfoot collapse and a short first MT. (*D, E*) Our fusion construct included the medial and middle columns. Allograft bone block lengthening of the first MT was also performed to restore medial column length and offload the lesser MT heads. A single extended incision in the first-second MT interspace was used. (*C*) After preparation of the first TMT joint space, a laminar spreader provides distraction and restoration of MT length and we monitor for signs of vascular compromise associated with overdistraction. (*D, E*) The appropriately sized structural allograft was fashioned and inserted. Plate fixation across the TMT articulations was chosen to increase stability of the fusion construction. Forefoot abduction was corrected with a lateral column lengthening (also using structural allograft). Z lengthening of the extensor hallucis longus tendon needs to be performed to prevent cock-up deformity of the hallux after medial column lengthening.

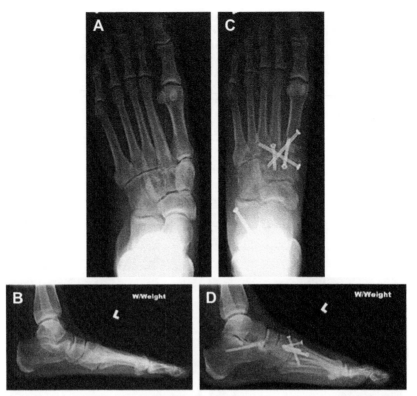

Fig. 4. Correction of abduction deformity. (*A, B*) This patient presented with symptomatic primary degenerative arthritis of the first and second TMT joints associated with a flexible pes planus deformity and forefoot abduction. First MT lengthening is not indicated because of asymptomatic bilateral brachymetatarsia. (*C, D*) Arthrodesis of the first and second TMT joints was performed through a single dorsal incision, using only screw fixation. To correct forefoot abduction, a lateral column lengthening through the anterior calcaneus was performed using structural allograft. Note that if a lateral soft tissue contracture prevents adequate correction of forefoot abduction, the peroneal brevis tendon is lengthened to allow additional correction.

stability as well as compression and the option for locking the screws. The ultimate decision regarding mode of fixation is dictated by the local anatomy, osteopenia, segmental bone loss, the joints to be fused, and perhaps, surgeon preference.

Plantar plate fixation of the medial column can be used in the settings of severe instability, when the fusion needs to be extended across the navicular-cuneiform joint, and when there is increased potential for nonunion (neuropathic arthropathy). When compared with a crossed screw configuration at the first TMT joint, application of a plantar one-third tubular plate on the tension side of the construct showed significantly higher load to failure.[11] Medial plate application has also been described for midfoot arthrodesis (**Fig. 6**). Horton and Olney[12] report reliable fusion results in patients who require salvage midfoot arthrodesis with residual correction of planovalgus, and cavovarus deformities.

The need to extend the fusion construct across the talonavicular joint poses a unique challenge. Plantar plate application, although biomechanically stronger

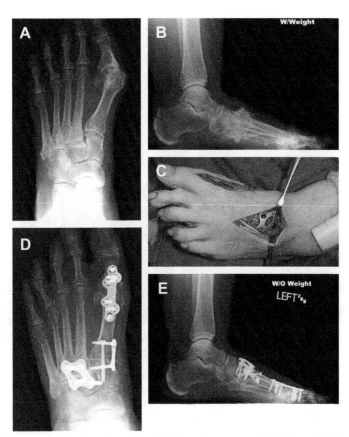

Fig. 5. Middle column fusion plate. (*A, B*) This patient presented with painful medial and middle column arthritis as well as a symptomatic hallux valgus deformity. (*C–E*) Midfoot arthrodesis included the symptomatic medial and middle columns and was accomplished through 2 longitudinal incisions, 1 medially over the first TMT joint and a second more lateral incision between the second and third TMT joints. Medial column fixation was performed first and included 1 axially placed partially threaded screw followed by a 2-hole OrthoLink plate (OrthoHelix, Medina, OH, USA). Note that a burr was used to create a well in the first MT cortex for the head of the screw. Next, a 4-hole Maxlock Extreme plate is used for middle column fixation. The plate is fixed proximally to the cuneiforms. Distal fixation then allows compression across the second and third TMT joints. The medial incision was extended dorsomedially to permit arthrodesis of the first MTP joint.

than a dorsomedial plate, is anatomically challenging. One alternative is to use a locking plate that is applied dorsally, medially, or dorsomedially. Locking plates provide fixed-angle stability and have been shown to be 4 times stronger than conventional plates.[13] They also provide improved fixation in osteoporotic bone.[14] As opposed to conventional plates, strength of the locking plate construct does not rely on friction generated by screw torque. Therefore, decreased compression and friction at the bone-plate interface preserve the periosteal blood supply[15] and may assist with healing. These qualities of locking plates also make them desirable for use in Charcot reconstruction, when bone loss, severe osteopenia, and dysvascularity make realignment and stable fixation technically difficult.

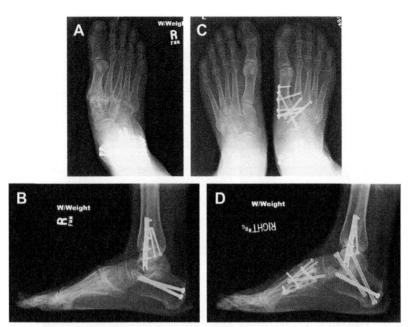

Fig. 6. Painful posttraumatic arthritis. (*A, B*) Radiographs reveal significant arthrosis throughout the midfoot, with an unstable short medial column. (*C, D*) The decision was made to include the entire medial and middle columns in the fusion construct. The lateral column was excluded to retain motion. A 2-incision approach was used with 1 midline medial incision and 1 dorsal incision centered between the second and third MTs. Joint space preparation further shortened the medial column and necessitated the use of structural allograft to maintain preoperative medial column length. A medial plate was chosen to supplement 1 retrograde screw across the first TMT joint. Screws placed through the plate extend into the middle column to further stabilize the construct.

Fixation in Charcot arthropathy can also be accomplished with intramedullary techniques. Sammarco and colleagues[16] reported their results after axial placement of intramedullary screws in 22 patients with Charcot arthropathy. Complete union occurred in 73% of 22 patients at a mean of 6 months. There were no amputations and all patients were ambulatory within 10 months. These investigators acknowledge that their technique crosses joints not involved in the fusion construct, and that motion at these joints may lead to screw migration and breakage. They further recommend not crossing an uninvolved talonavicular joint unless absolutely necessary. Benefits of this technique include fewer stress risers in cortical bone, more limited incisions without extensive soft tissue stripping, and diminished concern for exposed hardware in the event of wound breakdown.[17] Another intramedullary fixation system is available; use of the TARSX system (Extremity Medical, Parsippany, NJ, USA) for reconstruction of a Charcot foot is illustrated in **Fig. 7**. Note the extensive osteopenia and midfoot fragmentation, dorsal dislocation of the forefoot, and lateral rocker bottom deformity. The MT implants are inserted sequentially in antegrade fashion over a guide wire. The lag screws are then inserted retrogradely through the proximal edge of the MT implant and are considered seated when engaged in the Morse taper of the MT implant.

A final case example illustrates many of the principles discussed earlier for the correction of midfoot arthritis and deformity. The patient presented with a painful

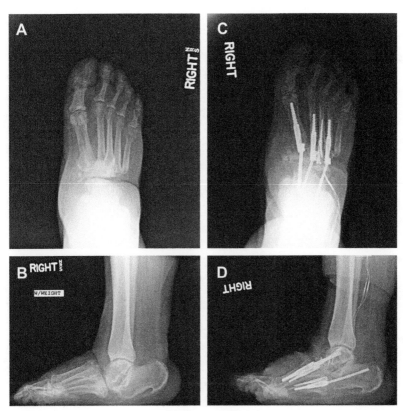

Fig. 7. Intermedullary fixation. (*A, B*) Radiographs show extensive fragmentation and collapse associated with a Charcot arthropathy. (*C, D*) The TARSX system was used for reconstruction and fusion. We typically approach this deformity using a 3-incision technique: 1 midline medial incision and 2 dorsal incisions in the interspaces between the second and third MTs and the fourth and fifth MTs. The same principles apply: start with the medial column and move stepwise laterally. We had difficulty properly cannulating the third MT and chose to forego placing the proximal lag screw. The implant was left in the third MT to avoid iatrogenic injury with attempted extraction. A bone stimulator was implanted to encourage successful arthrodesis, which is essential to maintain correction after realignment.

neuropathic arthropathy. Radiographs (**Fig. 8**) reveal fragmentation and collapse through the midfoot with lateral subluxation of the middle and lateral columns and associated forefoot abduction and hindfoot valgus. Realignment is required, and all 3 columns need to be included in the arthrodesis. Realignment started with a medial-izing calcaneal osteotomy to correct hindfoot valgus. Realignment was accomplished before inflating the tourniquet. A standard 3-incision approach was then used. Wedge resection was not performed to prevent shortening. Midfoot realignment started with the medial column after joint space preparation of all 3 columns. With the hallux dorsi-flexed, reduction of the first TMT joint was accomplished with axial pressure along the first MT combined with slight adduction. Provisional reduction consisted of a single guide wire for a 4-mm cannulated screw inserted from the dorsal aspect of the first

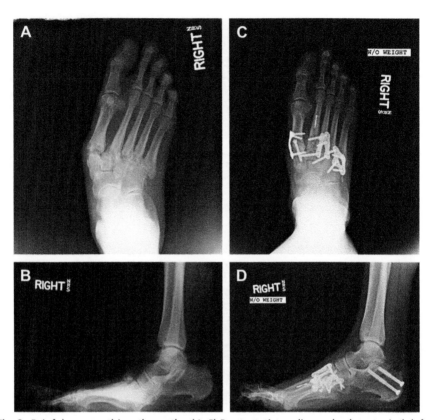

Fig. 8. Painful neuropathic arthropathy. (*A, B*) Preoperative radiographs show typical deformity associated with a Charcot arthropathy, including hindfoot valgus, midfoot collapse, and forefoot abduction. (*C, D*) Postoperative radiographs confirm adequate restoration of the talus-first MT line in both the anterior-posterior and lateral radiographs as well as restoration of the longitudinal arch and MT declination angle.

MT into the medial cuneiform. The middle and lateral columns were then rotated medially against a stable medial column and provisionally fixed with K-wires. Definitive fixation of the fusion construct started with the medial column as well. One partially threaded cannulated screw was placed retrograde from the first MT into the medial cuneiform after using the burr to create a well for the screw head. A medial plate was applied across the first TMT joint to complete the fusion construct of the medial column. Given the poor bone quality and fragmentation, plate fixation was also used to secure the middle and lateral columns. Compression across the second and third TMT joints was obtained using 2- and 3-hole OrthoLink (OrthoHelix, Medina, OH, USA) plates, respectively. A 4-hole Maxlock Extreme (OrthoHelix, Medina, OH, USA) plate was used for fixation of the lateral column. Postoperative radiographs show adequate restoration of alignment.

Proper realignment and successful arthrodesis are essential for durable correction of deformity. Once the initial decisions have been made regarding the need for realignment and which joints to include in the arthrodesis, the surgical plan should take into account surgical approach, joint space preparation, order of fixation, and choice of fixation constructs. In addition, for the correction of severe deformity associated with neuropathic arthropathy, realignment may need to incorporate techniques including wedge resection, lateral column arthrodesis, medial plantar plating, the use of locking plate constructs, and intermedullary fixation.

REFERENCES

1. Davitt JS, Kadel N, Sangeorzan BJ, et al. An association between functional second metatarsal length and midfoot arthrosis. J Bone Joint Surg Am 2005; 87:795–800.
2. Schepers T, Kieboom B, van Diggele P, et al. Pedobarographic analysis and quality of life after Lisfranc fracture dislocation. Foot Ankle Int 2010;31(10): 857–64.
3. Jung HG, Myerson MS, Schon LC. Spectrum of operative treatments and clinical outcomes for atraumatic osteoarthritis of the tarsometatarsal joints. Foot Ankle Int 2007;28(4):482–9.
4. Sangeorzan BJ, Veith RG, Hansen ST. Salvage of Lisfranc's tarsometatarsal joint by arthrodesis. Foot Ankle 1990;10:193–200.
5. Komenda GA, Myerson MS, Biddinger KR. Results of arthrodesis of the tarsome-tatarsal joints after traumatic injury. J Bone Joint Surg Am 1996;78:1665–76.
6. Den Hartog BD, Kay DB. Non-neuropathic midfoot multiplanar deformity: surgical strategies for reconstruction. Foot Ankle Clin 2009;14:383–92.
7. Ouzounian TJ, Shereff MJ. In vitro determination of midfoot motion. Foot Ankle 1989;10:140–6.
8. Raikin SM, Schon LC. Arthrodesis of the fourth and fifth tarsometatarsal joints of the midfoot. Foot Ankle Int 2003;24(8):584–90.
9. Vertullo CJ, Easley ME, Nunley JA. The transverse dorsal approach to the Lis-franc joint. Foot Ankle Int 2002;23(5):420–6.
10. Myerson MS, Neufeld SK, Uribe J. Fresh-frozen structural allografts in the foot and ankle. J Bone Joint Surg Am 2005;87:113–20.
11. Marks RM, Parks BG, Schon LC. Midfoot fusion technique for neuroarthropathic feet: biomechanical analysis and rationale. Foot Ankle Int 1998;19(8):507–10.
12. Horton GA, Olney BW. Deformity correction and arthrodesis of the midfoot with a medial plate. Foot Ankle 1993;14(9):493–9.
13. Gautier E, Sommers C. Guidelines for the clinical application of the LCP. Injury 2003;34:B63–76.
14. Haidukewych GJ, Ricci W. Locked plating in orthopaedic trauma: a clinical update. J Am Acad Orthop Surg 2008;16(6):347–55.
15. Farouk O, Krettek T, Miclau T. Minimally invasive plate osteosynthesis and vascu-larity: preliminary results of a cadaver injection study. Injury 1997;28:A7–12.
16. Sammarco VJ, Sammarco GJ, Walker EW, et al. Midtarsal arthrodesis in the treat-ment of Charcot midfoot arthropathy. J Bone Joint Surg Am 2009;91:80–91.
17. Sammarco VJ. Superconstructs in the treatment of Charcot foot deformity: plantar plating, locked plating, and axial screw fixation. Foot Ankle Clin 2009;19: 393–407.

The Isolated Talonavicular Arthrodesis

Xavier Crevoisier, MD, PD

KEYWORDS

• Chopart joint • Talonavicular joint • Talonavicular arthrodesis

Isolated talonavicular arthrodesis is performed to correct deformities of the hindfoot and treat degenerative, inflammatory, or posttraumatic disorders of the talonavicular joint. This procedure is known to provide significant functional improvement despite its major consequences on the residual motion of the hindfoot.

Most literature reports deal with disorders and deformities in adults, but in a review article, Weinheimer[1] stated that isolated talonavicular fusion was originally described by Ogston[2] in 1884 for children with severe pronated feet.

This article presents an overview of the indications, operative techniques, biomechanical consequences, and results associated with this procedure and discusses the relationship between the pathologic conditions treated and the obtained results. The value of the existing literature and the need for further investigation are also examined.

INDICATIONS

Isolated talonavicular arthrodesis has been described for the following indications:

- Hindfoot stabilization in cases of early valgus deformity of the hindfoot in rheumatoid arthritis (RA)[3]
- Flexible flatfoot deformity secondary to posterior tibial tendon dysfunction (**Fig. 1**)[3–7]
- Isolated posttraumatic arthritis,[3,8] primary arthritis,[8,9] or RA[10–12] of the talonavicular joint (**Fig. 2**)
- Equinovarus deformity in neurologic disorders[3]
- Paralytic postpoliomyelitis condition[13]
- Pes planus valgus in children and adolescents with cerebral palsy[14]
- Dorsal subluxation of the navicular in resistant clubfoot.[15,16]

The author has nothing to disclose.
Department of Orthopedic Surgery, Centre Hospitalier Universitaire Vaudois (CHUV), Site Hôpital Orthopédique, CH-1011 Lausanne, Switzerland
E-mail address: xavier.crevoisier@chuv.ch

Foot Ankle Clin N Am 16 (2011) 49–59
doi:10.1016/j.fcl.2010.11.002
1083-7515/11/$ – see front matter © 2011 Elsevier Inc. All rights reserved.

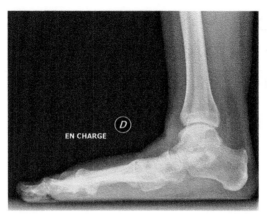

Fig. 1. Lateral radiograph of the weight-bearing right foot showing flattening of the longitudinal arch as seen in flexible flatfoot deformity secondary to posterior tibial tendon dysfunction.

In case of flatfoot or cavus foot deformity, a lengthening of the Achilles tendon may be added to the procedure.[3]

SURGICAL TECHNIQUE

The surgical approaches for isolated talonavicular arthrodesis include a medial incision between the tibialis posterior and the tibialis anterior (TA) tendons,[3,5–7,12,17–19] a dorsomedial incision just medial to the TA tendon,[4,8,11,20] and a dorsal incision between the TA and the extensor hallucis longus (EHL) tendons[21] or even between the EHL and the extensor digitorum longus tendons.[22]

Several fixation techniques have been described: compression screw fixation (**Fig. 3**),[4–6,8,10,18,23] staple fixation (**Fig. 4**),[8,9,12,18,20] combination of compression screw and staple fixation,[11,17,18] simple[24] or locking[7] plate fixation, and combination of plate and compression screw fixation.[22,24] In an in vitro biomechanical study, Jarrell and colleagues[24] found little difference in the primary talonavicular stability between screw and plate-screw constructs. Fixation can be performed with[5,10,12,19,20,22] or without[8,18] bone grafting. Bone grafting can be simply achieved by interposition of cancellous bone chips, but some investigators have described subtle constructs including creation of a slot for insertion of a bridging bone plug or dowel.[19,20] If a dowel arthrodesis is

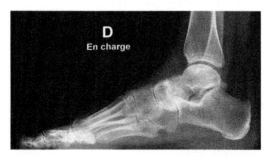

Fig. 2. Lateral radiograph of the weight-bearing right foot showing isolated talonavicular arthritis without deformation of the foot as is frequently observed in RA.

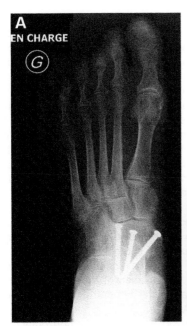

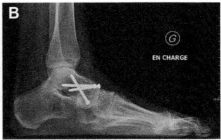

Fig. 3. Anteroposterior (*A*) and lateral (*B*) radiographs of the weight-bearing left foot showing consolidation of the talonavicular joint after 4.0-mm compression screw fixation.

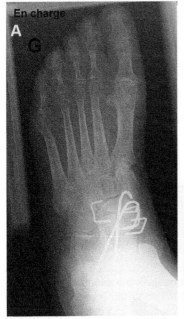

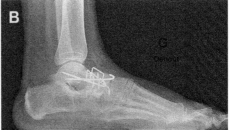

Fig. 4. Anteroposterior (*A*) and lateral (*B*) radiographs of the weight-bearing left foot showing nonunion of the talonavicular joint after combined staple and K-wire fixation.

performed, autogenous bone should be preferred to defatted bank bone.[25] To enhance both the primary stability and the contact area of the fused joint, most investigators recommend appreciating the concavity/convexity of the joint[3–5,8,10,17]; this process can also be achieved by transecting the talus and navicular into congruent positive-negative shapes.[21]

The procedure is easy in case of in situ fusion for isolated talonavicular arthritis but very demanding in case of acquired planovalgus deformity. As described by Fortin,[4] the navicular can be medialized easily, but this correction frequently supinates the forefoot. At this point, care must be taken to simultaneously plantarize the navicular, but this process may result in incongruency of the joint reduction and necessitate cancellous bone grafting. In some patients, despite adequate positioning of the talonavicular arthrodesis, medial column support remains insufficient and results in a functional supinatus of the forefoot, and in this case, additional plantarizing fusion of the first cuneometatarsal joint may be necessary.

In the past, at the author's institution, the medial approach was preferred because the position in the sagittal plane was thought to be controlled more accurately, especially in case of acquired flatfoot deformity. At present, a dorsal incision between the TA and EHL tendons is preferred (**Fig. 5**A, B). Lateral retraction of the EHL tendon protects the arteria dorsalis pedis and allows visualization of the lateral aspect of the talonavicular joint (see **Fig. 5**C), providing an excellent control of the position in the horizontal plane. Medial retraction of the TA tendon allows exposition of the dorsomedial and medial aspects of the joint line, providing control in the horizontal plane and in the sagittal plane as well. Then, a Hintermann distractor is used for exposition of the joint surfaces (see **Fig. 5**D). The cartilage is removed using a sharp chisel (see **Fig. 5**E), and the concavity/convexity of the joint is preserved to maintain a large contact area. To promote fusion, multiple drilling into the subchondral bone is performed (see **Fig. 5**F), and a kind of fish scaling is created through microfracturing of the subchondral bone with a sharp osteotome (see **Fig. 5**G). Autologous cancellous bone grafting is performed (see **Fig. 5**H) if the talar and navicular surfaces do not adapt perfectly. Provisory fixation of the joint is achieved through threaded Kirschner (K) wires (see **Fig. 5**I); fluoroscopic control is performed, and cannulated compression screws are inserted over these K wires (see **Fig. 5**J). The author's approach allows insertion of the compression screws into the transverse area of the joint, and if a simultaneous plantar-medial compression is needed, a percutaneous screw insertion (see **Fig. 5**I) into the plantar-medial tuberosity of the navicular is easy. Double-threaded compression screws are used not only to achieve higher initial compression but also to avoid conflict of the head of the screw with the neighbor joints (**Fig. 6**).

POSTOPERATIVE CARE

Most investigators recommend a postoperative cast stabilization including 6 weeks of partial weight bearing followed by 6 weeks of progressive weight bearing depending on the radiological results at 6 weeks.[3–5,9–12,21]

BIOMECHANICAL CONSEQUENCES
In Vitro Analysis

Astion and colleagues[26] simulated isolated arthrodesis of the talonavicular, calcaneocuboid, or subtalar joints; double arthrodesis of the talonavicular and calcaneocuboid joints; and triple arthrodesis of the subtalar, talonavicular, and calcaneocuboid joints in 10 fresh frozen cadaveric foot specimen. They studied the pronation and supination of the foot and measured the range of motion of each joint not involved in the

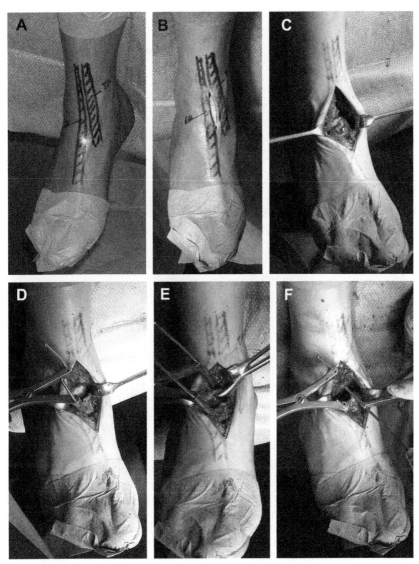

Fig. 5. Intraoperative views of an isolated talonavicular arthrodesis performed through a dorsal approach. The TA and EHL tendons are identified (*A*), and a longitudinal incision is performed between them (*B*). The joint line is exposed by medial retraction of the TA and lateral retraction of the EHL (*C*), and the surfaces are exposed using a distractor (*D*). The cartilage is removed using a sharp chisel (*E*), and then the subchondral bone is stimulated by multiple drilling (*F*) and microfracturing (*G*). Cancellous bone graft is inserted (*H*), provisory fixation is achieved through threaded K wires (*I*), and fluoroscopic control is used. Eventually, double-threaded compression screws are inserted over the K wires (*J*).

arthrodesis using a magnetic space tracking system (Fastrak; Polhemus Navigational Sciences Division, Colchester, VT, USA). Furthermore, they measured the excursion of the tibialis posterior tendon under these conditions and found that any arthrodesis involving the talonavicular joint essentially eliminates the motion of the other joints in the hindfoot complex and limits the excursion of the posterior tibial tendon to

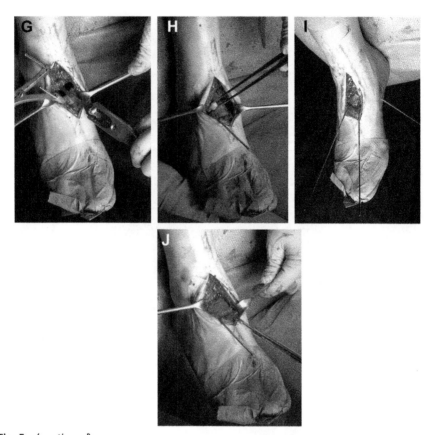

Fig. 5. (*continued*)

25% of the preoperative value. They concluded that the talonavicular joint, which has a physiologic mean range of motion of 37°, is the key joint of the hindfoot complex. This conclusion was confirmed in another similar study using an ultrasonic positioning system and loading the foot in flexion, extension, pronation, and supination, which was published in 2 different journals.[27,28] The conclusion obtained is also consistent with that of another previous in vitro study, conducted by O'Malley and colleagues,[29] comparing the efficacy of selected hindfoot arthrodeses to correct acquired flatfoot deformity. Thelen and colleagues[30] demonstrated that isolated talonavicular arthrodesis leads to a residual tarsal bone motion equivalent to that after double arthrodesis (talonavicular and calcaneocuboid) and that both the procedures provide the midtarsal and subtalar joints with comparable biomechanical stability. The suggested clinical relevance of this in vitro study is that isolated talonavicular arthrodesis is an effective alternative to double arthrodesis because it is less invasive, less complicated, and functionally equivalent. Nevertheless, a different conclusion was obtained by Thomas and colleagues[31] who examined the effect of these 2 procedures on subtalar contact and pressure and suggested that double arthrodesis should be preferred to talonavicular arthrodesis.

Isolated talonavicular arthrodesis is also associated with modified kinematics and kinetics at or proximal to the ankle joint. Hintermann and Nigg[32] examined the effects of selected hindfoot arthrodeses on the tibial rotation during flexion-extension of the

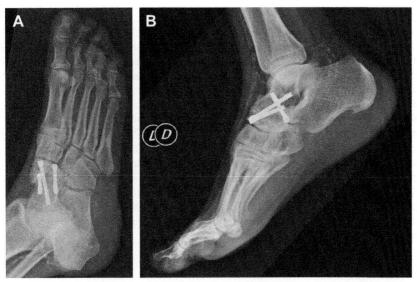

Fig. 6. Postoperative oblique (*A*) and lateral (*B*) radiographs of the right foot showing isolated fixation of the talonavicular joint with double-threaded compression screws. Note that 1 screw has been inserted from plantar-medial to dorsolateral direction to enhance plantar compression of the joint.

foot and found that isolated talonavicular arthrodesis increased the tibial rotation much less than tibiotalar arthrodesis. Suckel and colleagues[33] demonstrated that isolated talonavicular arthrodesis resulted in a lower and more evenly distributed peak pressure load in the ankle joint than triple arthrodesis. The suggested clinical relevance of this in vitro study is that when isolated talonavicular arthrodesis is a differential indication for triple arthrodesis, the former should be preferred to the latter.

In Vivo Analysis

Fishco and Cornwall[34] performed gait analysis before and after talonavicular arthrodesis for correction of flatfoot deformity. They found a reduced contact area in the medial longitudinal arch of the foot, a 70% reduction in total hindfoot inversion, and an increased time of heel-off during the stance phase of gait, from 45% to 83%. Although the study was limited to 2 patients (3 feet), the investigators emphasized the stabilizing effect of isolated talonavicular fusion on the hindfoot, and their results are consistent with the in vitro findings reported by Astion and colleagues.[26] Using a triaxial electrogoniometer, Fogel and colleagues[9] compared 6 patients who underwent talonavicular arthrodesis with 8 normal subjects and found decreased step length and reduced velocity in patients with talonavicular fusion. The total hindfoot coronal motion was reduced to approximately 73% that of the normal subjects, which is a much less reduction of motion than that reported in the biomechanical studies of Astion and colleagues[26] and Fishco and Cornwall.[34]

CLINICAL RESULTS

Most series report significant pain relief, satisfaction, and functional improvement after isolated talonavicular arthrodesis for several indications.

Results of Isolated Talonavicular Arthritis and RA

A significant increase of the American Orthopaedic Foot and Ankle Society (AOFAS) score from 77 to 93 was reported in a series of 16 patients with isolated talonavicular arthritis.[8] In another series of 26 patients with RA with isolated talonavicular arthritis and posterior tibial tendon dysfunction, an increase of the preoperative AOFAS score from 48 to 89 was reported.[18] The same conclusion, according to different outcome tools, was achieved in another study assessing 12 patients with RA with isolated talonavicular arthritis independent of flexible flatfoot deformity.[10] In another series of 17 patients with similar indications, Ljung and colleagues[20] reported 100% pain relief despite achievement of osseous union in only 12 feet. Elbar and colleagues[12] evaluated 35 isolated talonavicular fusions (26 cases of RA and 9 cases of osteoarthritis) and found complete relief of hindfoot pain in 75% of cases and mild improvement in 11% of cases; there was also an 89% satisfaction rate directly associated with improved ambulation. In a long-term (9.5 years) follow-up study, Fogel and colleagues[9] reported 100% satisfactory pain relief, but all patients experienced difficulty during ambulation on irregular grounds.

Results of Flexible Flatfoot Deformity

There are few studies focusing on the use of isolated talonavicular arthrodesis for flexible flatfoot deformity secondary to posterior tibial tendon dysfunction. Harper[5] assessed 29 patients, with an average follow-up of 2 years. The satisfaction rate was 86%, and the most common cause of reservation was lateral midfoot pain in the sinus tarsi. The objective evaluation of the results included the assessment of fusion, pain or instability, gait and function, and the absence of deformity or callosities. According to these criteria, the results were excellent in 11 patients, good in 14 patients, and fair in only 4 patients. In a series of 50 patients with isolated talonavicular arthrodesis, Asencio and colleagues[3] included only 3 patients with acquired flatfoot deformity secondary to posterior tibial tendon dysfunction but concluded that this procedure is adequate for treating flexible acquired flatfoot deformity. They also recommended to explore the need for Achilles tendon lengthening as an additional procedure. In a publication discussing the patient selection, the surgical technique, and a nonfocused review of the literature, Fortin[4] suggested that isolated talonavicular fusion may be used as an alternative to triple arthrodesis for treating flexible flatfoot deformity secondary to posterior tibial tendon dysfunction.

Results of Residual Deformities of a Previously Corrected Clubfoot

Painful dorsolateral subluxation and degenerative changes of the talonavicular joint with consecutive cavus deformity of the forefoot are the well-known consequences of surgically treated clubfoot deformity. Wei and colleagues[16] and Swaroop and colleagues[15] reported series of 16 and 13 patients, respectively. Both the studies found a 90% satisfaction rate associated with complete pain relief and also noted significant improvement in the talo-first metatarsal angle.

COMPLICATIONS

Nonunion has been reported in 0% to 35% of patients.[3,5,6,8,10–12,17,18,20] In case of isolated talonavicular arthritis in RA without deformity of the hindfoot, compression screw arthrodesis in combination with autologous bone grafting has been shown to reduce the nonunion rate to 0% to 5%.[10,17]

Development or progression of arthritic changes in the neighbor joints after isolated talonavicular arthrodesis occurs in up to 30% to 37% of patients[5,6,8,9,12,20,22] but does not seem to affect the clinical outcome.[8]

Complex regional pain syndrome may occur in 0% to 18% of patients.[3,8]

The deep infection rate ranges from 0% to 2%,[3,8,12] whereas superficial wound infection or scar dehiscence occurs in 0% to 10% of patients.[5,9,11,18]

DISCUSSION

As mentioned earlier, the overall results of talonavicular arthrodesis have been reported to be good or excellent. Nevertheless, the quality and heterogeneity of the literature reports related to this technique should be known. To the best of the author's knowledge, no prospective trial differentiating the indications has been conducted and reported. Furthermore, most retrospective studies are poorly conducted. In fact, there are major issues regarding the methodology for patient selection, the operative technique, and the assessment of the results. Eventually, most series include small numbers of patients, with short follow-up periods. Therefore, in the author's opinion, at present, no definitive conclusion can be withdrawn from the existing literature. However, the literature about isolated talonavicular arthrodesis includes strong biomechanical evaluations, which may serve as an excellent basis for further prospective trials.

Despite these statements, the existing literature, at least, provides some important trends related to isolated talonavicular arthrodesis. In case of RA, which was the most studied condition, isolated talonavicular arthrodesis seemed to be a nonextensive procedure that provides excellent pain relief and prevents further deformity of the hindfoot and, therefore, eliminates the need for more elaborate corrective surgery.[10,12,17,18,20] This result seems to be true also for isolated arthritis of the talonavicular joint, assuming that a stable primary fixation is achieved using compression screws or their combination with plates or staples. There are few studies about the correction of flexible acquired flatfoot by talonavicular fusion, but this procedure seems to be a valuable alternative to more invasive procedures. However, performing talonavicular arthrodesis to correct a deformity is much more demanding than fusing the joint in situ.[4] There are 2 small series focusing on the use of the procedure to treat painful dorsolateral subluxation of the talonavicular joint after the clubfoot deformity is treated surgically. The results regarding pain relief and morphologic correction are uniform; therefore, talonavicular arthrodesis can be recommended for this indication.

Gait analysis has shown that, even if significant pain relief and functional improvement can be achieved by talonavicular arthrodesis, patients may experience difficulty during ambulation on irregular surfaces,[9] which is because of the important locking of the hindfoot joint complex by the sole talonavicular arthrodesis, a fact that has also been clearly established in vitro.[26–28]

SUMMARY

Isolated talonavicular arthrodesis seems to be an efficient procedure to treat deformities of the hindfoot and degenerative, inflammatory, or posttraumatic disorders of the talonavicular joint. This procedure leads to significant pain relief and functional improvement in these pathologic conditions. Talonavicular arthrodesis for correction of hindfoot deformities is technically more demanding than in situ arthrodesis of the talonavicular joint. Compression screw fixation with or without plates or staples provides the most efficient primary stability and decreases the nonunion rate associated with this procedure. Biomechanical studies have demonstrated the key role of the talonavicular joint in the complex mobility of the hindfoot. There is a need for prospective studies associated with rigorous methodology to confirm the results reported by retrospective studies including small numbers of patients and short follow-up periods.

REFERENCES

1. Weinheimer D. Talonavicular arthrodesis. Clin Podiatr Med Surg 2004;21:227.
2. Ogston A. On flatfoot and its cure by operation. BMJ 1884;9:110.
3. Asencio G, Roeland A, Megy B, et al. [Stabilization of the hindfoot by talonavicular arthrodesis. Results apropos of 50 cases]. Rev Chir Orthop Reparatrice Appar Mot 1995;81:691 [in French].
4. Fortin PT. Posterior tibial tendon insufficiency. Isolated fusion of the talonavicular joint. Foot Ankle Clin 2001;6:137.
5. Harper MC. Talonavicular arthrodesis for the acquired flatfoot in the adult. Clin Orthop Relat Res 1999;365:65–8.
6. Mothershed RA, Stapp MD, Smith TF. Talonavicular arthrodesis for correction of posterior tibial tendon dysfunction. Clin Podiatr Med Surg 1999;16:501.
7. Weinraub GM, Heilala MA. Isolated talonavicular arthrodesis for adult onset flatfoot deformity/posterior tibial tendon dysfunction. Clin Podiatr Med Surg 2007;24:745.
8. Chen CH, Huang PJ, Chen TB, et al. Isolated talonavicular arthrodesis for talonavicular arthritis. Foot Ankle Int 2001;22:633.
9. Fogel GR, Katoh Y, Rand JA, et al. Talonavicular arthrodesis for isolated arthrosis: 9.5-year results and gait analysis. Foot Ankle 1982;3:105.
10. Carl HD, Pfander D, Weseloh G, et al. [Talonavicular arthrodesis for the rheumatoid foot]. Z Rheumatol 2006;65:633 [in German].
11. Chiodo CP, Martin T, Wilson MG. A technique for isolated arthrodesis for inflammatory arthritis of the talonavicular joint. Foot Ankle Int 2000;21:307.
12. Elbar JE, Thomas WH, Weinfeld MS, et al. Talonavicular arthrodesis for rheumatoid arthritis of the hindfoot. Orthop Clin North Am 1976;7:821.
13. Faraj AA. Talonavicular joint arthrodesis for paralytic post poliomyelitis forefoot instability. J Foot Ankle Surg 1996;35:166.
14. Turriago CA, Arbelaez MF, Becerra LC. Talonavicular joint arthrodesis for the treatment of pes planus valgus in older children and adolescents with cerebral palsy. J Child Orthop 2009;3:179.
15. Swaroop VT, Wenger DR, Mubarak SJ. Talonavicular fusion for dorsal subluxation of the navicular in resistant clubfoot. Clin Orthop Relat Res 2009;467:1314.
16. Wei SY, Sullivan RJ, Davidson RS. Talo-navicular arthrodesis for residual midfoot deformities of a previously corrected clubfoot. Foot Ankle Int 2000;21:482.
17. Kindsfater K, Wilson MG, Thomas WH. Management of the rheumatoid hindfoot with special reference to talonavicular arthrodesis. Clin Orthop Relat Res 1997;340:69–74.
18. Popelka S, Hromadka R, Vavrik P, et al. Isolated talonavicular arthrodesis in patients with rheumatoid arthritis of the foot and tibialis posterior tendon dysfunction. BMC Musculoskelet Disord 2010;11:38.
19. Potter TA. Talonavicular fusion with bone graft for spastic arthritic flat foot. Surg Clin North Am 1969;49:883.
20. Ljung P, Kaij J, Knutson K, et al. Talonavicular arthrodesis in the rheumatoid foot. Foot Ankle 1992;13:313.

21. Gould N. Technique tips: footings. Arthrodesis–talonavicular joint. Foot Ankle 1985;6:153.
22. Rammelt S, Marti RK, Zwipp H. [Arthrodesis of the talonavicular joint]. Orthopade 2006;35:428 [in German].
23. Rosenfeld JF, Parks BG, Schon LC. Biomechanical investigation of optimal fixation of isolated talonavicular joint fusion. Am J Orthop (Belle Mead NJ) 2005; 34:445.
24. Jarrell SE 3rd, Owen JR, Wayne JS, et al. Biomechanical comparison of screw versus plate/screw construct for talonavicular fusion. Foot Ankle Int 2009;30:150.
25. Thoren K, Ljung P, Pettersson H, et al. Comparison of talonavicular dowel arthrodesis utilizing autogenous bone versus defatted bank bone. Foot Ankle 1993;14: 125.
26. Astion DJ, Deland JT, Otis JC, et al. Motion of the hindfoot after simulated arthrodesis. J Bone Joint Surg Am 1997;79:241.
27. Wulker N, Stukenborg C, Savory KM, et al. Hindfoot motion after isolated and combined arthrodeses: measurements in anatomic specimens. Foot Ankle Int 2000;21:921.
28. Savory KM, Wulker N, Stukenborg C, et al. Biomechanics of the hindfoot joints in response to degenerative hindfoot arthrodeses. Clin Biomech (Bristol, Avon) 1998;13:62.
29. O'Malley MJ, Deland JT, Lee KT. Selective hindfoot arthrodesis for the treatment of adult acquired flatfoot deformity: an in vitro study. Foot Ankle Int 1995;16:411.
30. Thelen S, Rutt J, Wild M, et al. The influence of talonavicular versus double arthrodesis on load dependent motion of the midtarsal joint. Arch Orthop Trauma Surg 2009;130:47–53.
31. Thomas JL, Moeini R, Soileau R. The effects on subtalar contact and pressure following talonavicular and midtarsal joint arthrodesis. J Foot Ankle Surg 2000; 39:78.
32. Hintermann B, Nigg BM. Influence of arthrodeses on kinematics of the axially loaded ankle complex during dorsiflexion/plantarflexion. Foot Ankle Int 1995; 16:633.
33. Suckel A, Muller O, Herberts T, et al. Talonavicular arthrodesis or triple arthrodesis: peak pressure in the adjacent joints measured in 8 cadaver specimens. Acta Orthop 2007;78:592.
34. Fishco WD, Cornwall MW. Gait analysis after talonavicular joint fusion: 2 case reports. J Foot Ankle Surg 2004;43:241.

Triple Arthrodesis

Markus Knupp, MD[a],*, Sjoerd A.S. Stufkens, MD[b],
Beat Hintermann, MD[c]

KEYWORDS

- Triple arthrodesis • Flatfoot deformity
- Posterior tibial tendon insufficiency • Hindfoot deformity

Triple arthrodesis traditionally consists of fusion of the talonavicular, calcaneocuboid, and subtalar joints, which are performed through a medial and lateral approach. Initially this procedure was used to treat the sequelae of paralytic disease.[1,2] The aim was to achieve a plantigrade foot that maintained stability in the frontal plane. As the number of patients with deformity due to paralysis declined, triple arthrodesis was performed less often. Later, the procedure regained popularity by its ability to restore a painful and deformed hindfoot, caused by residuals of trauma,[3] rheumatoid arthritis,[4,5] and long-standing posterior tibial tendon dysfunction.[6–8]

Although triple arthrodesis is a valuable tool for hindfoot correction, it is not without postoperative complications, including malunions and nonunions, lateral wound breakdown, and induction of adjacent joint osteoarthritis.[4–6,8,9] Therefore several modifications of the initial technique have been suggested. Sparing the calcaneocuboid joint, for example, isolated fusion of the talonavicular and the subtalar joint only, can achieve comparable good results in nonparalytic patients.[10] Advantages of this technique include reduction of the operative time and the risk of nonunion.[9,11] In addition, avoiding further shortening of the lateral column by not fusing the calcaneocuboid joint greatly facilitates reduction of the abducted foot.[12] Retention of the calcaneocuboid joint provides some movement[13] and thereby diminishes the loading on the adjacent joints, which may lead to osteoarthritis.[4–6,8,9]

In patients with severe flatfoot deformity correction, breakdown of the lateral wounds has been described in several studies.[4–6,8,9] Wound problems may arise if correction of the deformity leads to increased tension on the lateral side of the foot. A technique that makes use of a single medial incision reduces the risk of problems with wound healing, especially in patients with severe deformity of the deficient lateral skin.[10,14,15] The feasibility of triple arthrodesis through a single medial approach has

The authors have nothing to disclose.
[a] Department of Orthopaedic Surgery, Kantonsspital Liestal, Rheinstrasse 26, CH-4410 Liestal, Switzerland
[b] Department of Orthopaedic Surgery, Academic Medical Center, Meibergdreef 9, 1105 AZ Amsterdam, The Netherlands
[c] Clinic of Orthopaedic and Trauma Surgery, Kantonsspital Liestal, Rheinstrasse 26, CH-4410, Switzerland
* Corresponding author.
E-mail address: markus.knupp@ksli.ch

been shown in cadaver[16] and clinical studies.[12,15,17] Placing the incision medially has been shown to improve visualization and exposure of the transverse tarsal joint[12,16] and to allow good control of the position of the joints to be fused.[10,12,16] The improved visualization facilitates debridement of the joints without placing the posteromedial structures, especially the flexor hallucis longus tendon, at risk.[10,12]

Based on all of the earlier-mentioned considerations, the authors decided to modify the triple arthrodesis into a "diple" arthrodesis, subtalar and talonavicular arthrodesis through a single medial approach, whenever a proper indication emerges.

SURGICAL INDICATIONS

Numerous pathologic processes can lead to a painful and/or malaligned hindfoot. Classical indications for a triple arthrodesis include arthritis of the hindfoot (rheumatoid or posttraumatic),[3–5] end-stage posterior tibial tendon dysfunction,[6–8] and neuromuscular disease-mediated hindfoot deformities.[1,2] In a large majority of these problems, the traditional triple arthrodesis can be replaced by fusion of the talonavicular and the subtalar joint through a single medial incision.

The traditional medial and lateral approach is preferred over the diple arthrodesis in patients with severe arthritic changes in the calcaneocuboid joint and with severe cavovarus deformity in which the subtalar joint cannot be visualized properly form the medial side. Patients with a limited dorsiflexion in their ankle or a drop foot are

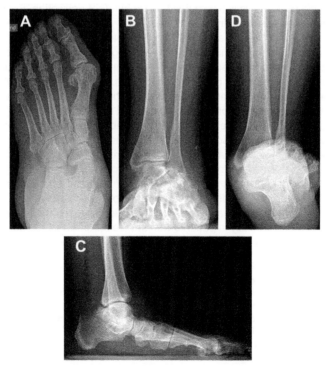

Fig. 1. Preoperative weight-bearing radiographs of a 65-year-old female patient with a long-standing stage III posterior tibial tendon insufficiency. (*A*) The dorsoplantar view shows talonavicular subluxation; (*B*) the mortise view, subfibular impingement; (*C*) the lateral view, flattening of the longitudinal arch; and (*D*) the Saltzman view, a lateralized calcaneal tuberosity.

considered for a Lambrinudi-type of triple arthrodesis.[18,19] In patients with sequelae of treated congenital clubfoot deformities,[20] hindfoot fusions should be avoided and the deformities addressed with corrective supramalleolar, calcaneal, or midfoot osteotomies.

PREOPERATIVE PLANNING

Preoperative planning includes a detailed history taking, a thorough clinical examination, and a review of the radiographs. Standing plain radiographs of the foot in the dorsoplantar (**Fig. 1**A) and lateral projections (see **Fig. 1**C) and standing mortise views of the ankle (see **Fig. 1**B) are indispensable. Before surgery, arthritic degeneration of the involved joints (and of the ankle and midfoot), global bone density, and/or intraosseous cysts must be taken into consideration. The authors routinely obtain a Saltzman hindfoot view (see **Fig. 1**D; **Fig. 2**).

SURGICAL TECHNIQUE

A 6-cm long skin incision is made from the navicular toward the medial malleolus, parallel to and approximately 5 mm above the posterior tibial tendon (**Fig. 3**). The

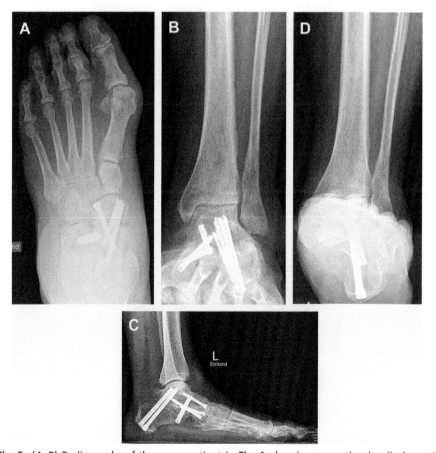

Fig. 2. (A–D) Radiographs of the same patient in **Fig. 1**, showing correction in all planes 1 year postoperation.

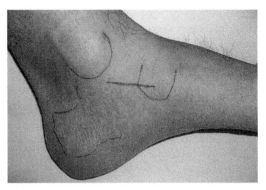

Fig. 3. Site of the incision.

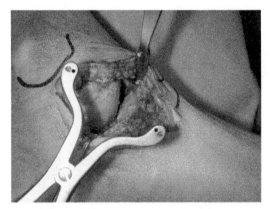

Fig. 4. Opening of the talonavicular joint.

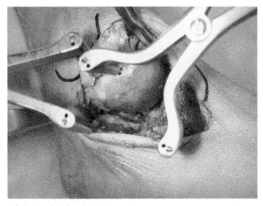

Fig. 5. Preparation of the subtalar joint.

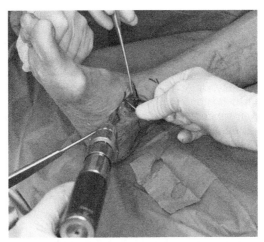

Fig. 6. Two K wires are used as "joysticks" to reduce the talonavicular joint (adduction and plantar flexion).

tendon sheath is opened and the tendon inspected. In cases with marked tendinosis, the tendon is excised. The capsule of the talonavicular joint is then incised. A spreader is placed dorsolaterally to open the talonavicular joint, which is subsequently denuded with a chisel (**Fig. 4**). Next, the calcaneal wall is exposed down to the sustentaculum. A Kirschner (K) wire is inserted into the base of the sustentaculum and then used to place the spreader over the talocalcaneal joint. Taking care not to damage the anterior fibers of the deltoid ligament, the subtalar joint is opened and denuded with a chisel and a curette and the exposed articular surfaces feathered or drilled with a 2-mm drill bit (**Fig. 5**). The foot is then held in a neutral position and K wires are used to secure the correction (**Figs. 6** and **7**). If the correction of the valgus deformity is insufficient,

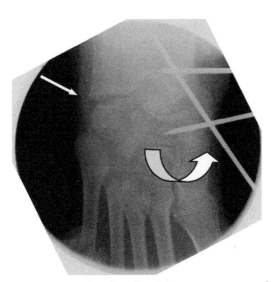

Fig. 7. Intraoperative radiograph showing the reduction maneuver of the talonavicular joint and the opening of the calcaneocuboid joint (*thin arrow*).

a medial displacement osteotomy of the calcaneus[21] is added before the subtalar joint is fused. For the osteotomy, an additional lateral approach is chosen.[12] Three cannulated compression screws for the talonavicular joint and 2 cannulated compression screws for the subtalar joint are used to achieve a stable fixation. In cases in which a calcaneal osteotomy is added, a second posterior screw is used to secure the tuberosity. Lengthening of the tendo Achillis is performed when a residual equinus position is present. Some investigators consider additional lengthening of the peroneal tendons.[14,15] Residual forefoot varus is addressed with a plantar flexion Cotton osteotomy (medial cuneiform).[22] A clinical example is shown in **Figs. 1** and **2**.

RESULTS

Sparing the calcaneocuboid joint did not adversely affect the outcome of the procedure[11,12] and reduction of the abducted forefoot was found to unload the calcaneocuboid joint.[12]

Reduction of wound healing problems caused by the single medial approach have been observed not only by the authors[10,12] but also in other reports.[14,15,17] Furthermore, the medial incision allows for an improved visualization and exposure of the transverse tarsal joints and thereby reduces the risk of malunions.[10,12,15,16]

SUMMARY

Triple arthrodesis originally has been used to treat the sequelae of paralytic disease and later became a very powerful procedure to address painful and/or malaligned hindfeet of different underlying pathologies. The extension of the original indication to the treatment of nonparalytic patients has led to the modification of the original technique to reduce the risk of postoperative complications. Limiting the triple arthrodesis to an isolated subtalar and talonavicular fusion, which can be performed through a single medial incision, can lead to equally good outcomes and therefore has become the preferred method for many surgeons. However, in patients with an underlying neurologic disease or severe cavovarus feet, the modified triple arthrodesis may not allow the stabilization and correction of the foot and the visualization of the joints may not be sufficient. In these cases, the traditional approach should be chosen.

REFERENCES

1. Ryerson. The classic. Arthrodesing operations on the feet: Edwin W. Ryerson, M.D. Clin Orthop Relat Res 1977;122:4–9.
2. Wetmore RS, Drennan JC. Long-term results of triple arthrodesis in Charcot-Marie-Tooth disease. J Bone Joint Surg Am 1989;71(3):417–22.
3. Klaue K. Chopart fractures. Injury 2004;35(Suppl 2):SB64–70.
4. Knupp M, Skoog A, Tornkvist H, et al. Triple arthrodesis in rheumatoid arthritis. Foot Ankle Int 2008;29(3):293–7.
5. Figgie MP, O'Malley MJ, Ranawat C, et al. Triple arthrodesis in rheumatoid arthritis. Clin Orthop Relat Res 1993;292:250–4.
6. Saltzman CL, Fehrle MJ, Cooper RR, et al. Triple arthrodesis: twenty-five and forty-four-year average follow-up of the same patients. J Bone Joint Surg Am 1999;81(10):1391–402.
7. Bennett GL, Graham CE, Mauldin DM. Triple arthrodesis in adults. Foot Ankle 1991;12(3):138–43.
8. Pell RF 4th, Myerson MS, Schon LC. Clinical outcome after primary triple arthrodesis. J Bone Joint Surg Am 2000;82(1):47–57.

9. Graves SC, Mann RA, Graves KO. Triple arthrodesis in older adults. Results after long-term follow-up. J Bone Joint Surg Am 1993;75(3):355–62.

10. DeWachter J, Knupp M, Hintermann B. Double-hindfoot arthrodesis through a single medial approach. Tech Foot Ankle Surg 2007;6:1–6.

11. Sammarco VJ, Magur EG, Sammarco GJ, et al. Arthrodesis of the subtalar and talonavicular joints for correction of symptomatic hindfoot malalignment. Foot Ankle Int 2006;27(9):661–6.

12. Knupp M, Schuh R, Stufkens SA, et al. Subtalar and talonavicular arthrodesis through a single medial approach for the correction of severe planovalgus deformity. J Bone Joint Surg Br 2009;91(5):612–5.

13. Astion DJ, Deland JT, Otis JC, et al. Motion of the hindfoot after simulated arthrodesis. J Bone Joint Surg Am 1997;79(2):241–6.

14. Jackson WF, Tryfonidis M, Cooke PH, et al. Arthrodesis of the hindfoot for valgus deformity. An entirely medial approach. J Bone Joint Surg Br 2007;89(7):925–7.

15. Jeng CL, Vora AM, Myerson MS. The medial approach to triple arthrodesis. Indications and technique for management of rigid valgus deformities in high-risk patients. Foot Ankle Clin 2005;10(3):515–21, vi–vii.

16. Jeng CL, Tankson CJ, Myerson MS. The single medial approach to triple arthrodesis: a cadaver study. Foot Ankle Int 2006;27(12):1122–5.

17. Brilhault J. Single medial approach to modified double arthrodesis in rigid flatfoot with lateral deficient skin. Foot Ankle Int 2009;30(1):21–6.

18. Wenz W, Bruckner T, Akbar M. Complete tendon transfer and inverse Lambrinudi arthrodesis: preliminary results of a new technique for the treatment of paralytic pes calcaneus. Foot Ankle Int 2008;29(7):683–9.

19. Elsner A, Barg A, Stufkens SA, et al. Lambrinudi arthrodesis with posterior tibialis transfer in adult drop-foot. Foot Ankle Int 2010;31(1):30–7.

20. Brodsky JW. The adult sequelae of treated congenital clubfoot. Foot Ankle Clin 2010;15(2):287–96.

21. Stufkens S, Knupp M, Hintermann B. Medial displacement calcaneal osteotomy. Tech Foot Ankle Surg 2009;8:85–90.

22. Cotton F. Foot statics and surgery. N Engl J Med 1936;214:353–62.

Subtalar and Naviculocuneiform Fusion for Extended Breakdown of the Medial Arch

Alexej Barg, MD[a,b,*], Samuel Brunner, MD[a], Lukas Zwicky, MSc[a],
Beat Hintermann, MD[c]

KEYWORDS

- Adult flatfoot deformity • Breakdown of medial arch
- Miller procedure
- Combined subtalar and naviculocuneiform fusion
- Medial column procedures in flatfoot deformity

Despite progress in understanding and treatment, the acquired flatfoot deformity remains a challenge for orthopedic surgeons. This situation is particularly true for the associated breakdown of the medial arch. Although a triple fusion is the most recommended surgical treatment option for stage III posterior tibial tendon dysfunction (PTTD),[1–6] it has limited correction of a fixed forefoot supinatus.[7] In particular, this treatment option is unable to compensate for breakdown at the naviculocuneiform (NC) and tarsometatarsal (TMT) joints (**Fig. 1**).

Inclusion of the NC joint in triple fusion theoretically permits more effective correction and improved stability at the medial arch and avoids a secondary break at the NC joint. Such an extended fusion may, however, significantly increase the load on distal joints and thus be a cause of the painful degenerative changes of adjacent joints often

This work was supported by research funding from Basel Foundation Orthopaedic Surgery and Biomechanics of Foot and Ankle (A.B.).
The authors have nothing to disclose.
[a] Clinic of Orthopaedic Surgery, Kantonsspital Liestal, Rheinstrasse 26, CH-4410 Liestal, Switzerland
[b] Harold K. Dunn Orthopaedic Research Laboratory, University Orthopaedic Center, 590 Wakara Way, Salt Lake City, UT 84108, USA
[c] Clinic of Orthopaedic and Trauma Surgery, Kantonsspital Liestal, Rheinstrasse 26, CH-4410, Switzerland
* Corresponding author. Clinic of Orthopaedic Surgery, Kantonsspital, Rheinstrasse 26, CH-4410 Liestal, Switzerland.
E-mail address: alexejbarg@mail.ru

Foot Ankle Clin N Am 16 (2011) 69–81
doi:10.1016/j.fcl.2010.11.004
1083-7515/11/$ – see front matter © 2011 Elsevier Inc. All rights reserved.

foot.theclinics.com

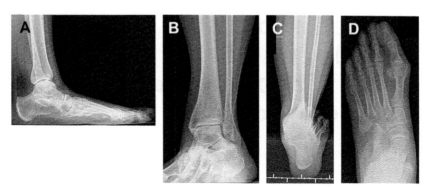

Fig. 1. Standard preoperative weight-bearing radiographs of a 63-year-old female patient with disabling PTTD and breakdown of the medial arch. (*A*) The lateral view shows a sag sign at the talonavicular (TN) and TMT joints and an increased talus–first metatarsal angle. (*B, C*) The anteroposterior (AP) view and the special hindfoot alignment view of the ankle show a significant valgus misalignment. (*D*) The AP view of the foot shows a subluxation at the TN joint with decreased navicular coverage and a decreased talus–first metatarsal angle.

reported after triple fusion.[8–11] Another conflicting problem that often presents in this patient cohort is an unstable first TMT joint and a severe valgus deformity at the first metatarsophalangeal joint. Therefore, we do not recommend extension of triple fusion to the NC joint because it stiffens the posterior aspect of the medial arch, overloads distal joints, and causes further breakdown. After such degeneration, fusion of the complete medial column may be the only way to salvage the foot.

After encountering this problem in some patients, we ended this strategy and began to consider another approach to stabilize the medial arch after extended breakdown. Subtalar (ST) fusion has been previously shown to be effective in addressing PTTD stage II or III flatfoot deformity if used with additional surgical options.[1,12–15] More than 80 years ago, Miller[16] reported a powerful correction of isolated NC fusion. Based on these findings, we established a rationale to combine ST fusion with NC fusion while preserving the talonavicular (TN) and calcaneocuboid (CC) joints. In this review article, we summarize the medial column procedures for flatfoot deformity and present our surgical technique and results of 10 consecutive patients treated with this method at a minimum 1-year follow-up.

MEDIAL COLUMN PROCEDURES IN FLATFOOT DEFORMITY
Miller Procedure

In 1927, Miller[16] published a clinical report describing a plastic flat foot operation correcting static flat foot in adolescent or preadolescent children. At that time, the flatfoot deformity was already recognized as a complex orthopedic problem. Miller developed a surgical technique for the correction of flexible (correctible) flatfoot deformity via fusion of the medial column (NC and first TMT fusion). In addition, the Achilles tendon was lengthened and an osteoperiosteal flap (on the insertion site of the calcaneonavicular ligament and posterior tibial tendon) was used to increase the stability of the restored medial arch. This surgical technique has been described as simple, short, and effective. In 16 adolescent patients at a midterm follow-up of 2.5 years, all reported a significant symptomatic improvement. Corrective loss of medial arch was not observed in any of the patients. Fraser and colleagues[17] studied the long-term results (mean follow-up was 12 years with a range between 3–27 years) of the

Miller procedure in 22 patients (38 feet). In 7 patients, the investigators modified the Miller procedure by adding a first TMT fusion. Of all the patients, 84% had satisfactory clinical outcomes, but a nonunion was observed in 21%. To our best knowledge, there are no peer-reviewed studies reporting the long-term results after the Miller procedure. This procedure was not recommended for patients with degenerative changes of the hindfoot joints and/or significant deformities at the TN and/or ST joints.

Hoke Procedure

While Miller[16] developed his surgical technique to address the flatfoot deformity in children and adolescents, Hoke[18] was the first to describe NC fusion in both adolescents and adults in 1931. Hoke analyzed the anatomic changes in patients with symptomatic flatfoot deformity and stated that the most critical aspects of the deformity were the contracted Achilles tendon and pathologically increased mobility of the midfoot joint, leading to breakdown of the medial arch. The surgical technique of Hoke[18] was similar to that described by Miller.[16] Hoke performed an open lengthening of the Achilles tendon followed by a bone-block fusion of the NC joint. The immediate postoperative casting of the foot in equinus position was reported as necessary to preserve the intraoperative correction of the medial arch. Between 1927 and 1934, Butte[19] performed the Hoke procedure in 138 patients. Butte found that higher age, obesity, increased laxity of midfoot, and progressive degenerative changes of midfoot were associated with worse outcomes. Jack[20] used the Hoke procedure to treat flatfoot deformity in 25 patients (46 feet) between 11 and 14 years of age. Jack introduced an anatomic classification for flatfoot deformities, distinguishing: (1) TN breaks (perpendicular talus), (2) NC breaks, and (3) combined breaks (both TN and NC joints are faulty). The midterm results with follow-up between 15 months and 5 years were satisfactory in 82% of all cases. However, Seymour[21] reported the long-term results (follow-up between 16 and 19 years) of 17 patients who were included in the study by Jack. The initial encouraging results were not maintained, with 50% of all patients unsatisfied with the results of surgery.

Modified Hoke-Miller Flatfoot Procedure

In 1983, Duncan and Lovell[22] published a clinical report describing a modification and combination of Miller[16] and Hoke[18] procedures. Their surgical technique included an NC fusion, an opening wedge osteotomy of the medial cuneiform, and a soft tissue procedure (distal advancement of an osteoperiosteal flap including the spring ligament). All 10 adolescent patients (17 feet) of this study reported postoperative improvement of symptoms at a minimum follow-up of 1 year. The subjects were able to perform all normal activities without restrictions. In general, results from this procedure are comparable to the Miller procedure.

Durham Flatfoot Plasty Procedure

In 1953, Caldwell[23] described a surgical technique to treat a symptomatic flexible flatfoot deformity. The surgery, originally introduced by Herbert Durham in 1935, was the combination of NC fusion with elevation of a ligamentous capsular flap and advancement of the posterior tibial tendon. At a mean follow-up of 6 years, most (94.7%) of the 38 patients enrolled in his study reported good or excellent results.

Isolated Medial Column Stabilization

Greisberg and colleagues[24] performed a midfoot arthrodesis (a modification of the Miller procedure[16]) for medial midfoot realignment in 19 patients with subluxation of the first TMT joint and/or significant sag at the medial NC joint. The main principle of their modified procedure, correction of deformity and rigid fixation, ensured long-term stability and rendered the additional soft tissue procedures and special postoperative casting techniques less important. Chi and colleagues[25] reviewed results of medial column stabilization, lateral column lengthening, and combined medial and lateral procedures in patients with adult acquired flatfoot deformity secondary to PTTD. Of the 5 patients, 4 with isolated medial column fusion were satisfied with the results of the surgery and had improved clinical symptoms. In general, this procedure is recommended in patients with PTTD stage II flatfoot deformity with residual forefoot deformity.[5] Coetzee and Hansen,[26] in contrast, also recommended this procedure in patients with PTTD stage III flatfoot deformity.

TN Fusion

Isolated fusion of the TN joint is another joint-preserving procedure for flatfoot correction.[27] The most common indication for this procedure is a painful unstable TN joint with fixed forefoot deformity. Patients with progressively painful degenerative changes of the ST should be excluded from this surgical procedure.[1] O'Malley and colleagues[28] have demonstrated in a biomechanical cadaver study that the TN fusion is able to sufficiently correct the flatfoot deformity through the transverse tarsal joint. However, the TN joint has the greatest range of motion of the triple joint complex, and fusion of this joint essentially eliminates the motion of the other joints of the complex.[29] These findings were confirmed by Fishco and Cornwall[30] using an electromagnetic motion analysis system. Furthermore, isolated TN fusion may increase and translate the pressure distribution of the ankle, ST joint, and remaining midfoot, resulting in painful degenerative changes.[27,31,32] Harper and Tisdel[32] performed isolated TN fusion in 27 consecutive patients with painful adult acquired flatfoot deformity. Excellent or good results were reported by 24 patients at the mean follow-up of 27 months. Progressive degenerative changes in adjacent joints were found in 5 patients. Three years later, Harper[33] reported the outcome of 29 patients who underwent isolated TN fusion with a mean follow-up of 26 months. In this study, 86% of all patients were satisfied with the procedures and reported good to excellent results. Recently, Camasta and colleagues[34] published a retrospective review of 51 TN joint fusions performed for flexible pes planovalgus deformity. In this study, 88% of all patients were satisfied with the procedure. However, the fusion rate was 100%. Six patients developed painful secondary osteoarthritis in adjacent joints: in 4 cases, the NC joint and in 2 cases, the ST joint. Therefore, patients should be carefully selected for isolated TN fusion. As suggested by Fortin,[27] the following concomitant deformities should be recognized and addressed when necessary: valgus deformity in combination with instability, degenerative changes of the ST and/or tibiotalar joint, and instability or collapse of the more distal midfoot joints.

INDICATIONS AND CONTRAINDICATIONS FOR ST AND NC FUSION

The most common indication for combined ST and NC fusion is the acquired adult stage III flatfoot deformity. Patients with this condition often present a significant breakdown of the medial arch (TN and/or NC joint) and report instability in the midtarsus during walking and/or standing. Most patients have forefoot varus deformity secondary to progressive PTTD. Also, the isolated breakdown of the medial arch without concomitant flatfoot deformity is another indication for this procedure.

The contraindications for this procedure are severe vascular and/or neurologic deficiency in the affected lower extremity. Also, this procedure should not be performed on heavy smokers because of the expected high rate of nonunion, as demonstrated in patients undergoing isolated ST arthrodesis.[35,36] The procedure should also not be considered for the treatment of Charcot neuroarthropathy. Relative contraindications are rheumatoid arthritis and advanced degenerative changes in the TN joint because they may progress and become more symptomatic after surgery.

PREOPERATIVE PLANNING
Clinical Examination

Preoperative planning begins with the careful assessment of patient history. The following aspects should be specifically addressed: actual pain, limitations in daily and sports activities, and current and previous treatments. All patients should be asked if they had trauma, concomitant diseases, infections, or surgeries in the past. Patients with any of the aforementioned contraindications should be excluded.

The routine physical examination includes careful inspection of both lower extremities and observation of the patient while walking and standing. The neurovascular status (pedal pulses and sensation) should be evaluated. In general, alignment, deformities, foot position, and muscular functioning/atrophy are assessed. In stage III flatfoot deformity, the medial longitudinal arch is significantly flattened (breakdown of the arch). Often, the talar head can be palpated medially as a prominent structure. The posterior tibial tendon is inspected and examined for pathologic conditions, such as thickening, warmth, soreness, and swelling. The strength of posterior tibial muscle can be proven by foot inversion against resistance in an everted and plantar flexed position. A simple sensitive sign of PTTD is the first metatarsal rise sign.[37,38] When the shank of the affected foot is taken with one hand and externally rotated or when the heel of the affected foot is taken with the other hand and brought passively into a varus position, the head of the first metatarsal rises in the case of PTTD and remains on the ground in normal posterior tibial function.[37] Furthermore, if the heel is in a valgus position, more toes are visible on the lateral side of the affected foot than on the contralateral side, which is called "too-many-toes sign."[1,38–40] However, this sign is absent in 20% to 35% of all cases.[37] All joints of the hindfoot and midfoot should be carefully assessed to determine which joints have reduced or absent motion and if these joints can be reduced (if irreducible, the deformity is then fixed).

Radiographic Evaluation

Radiographic evaluation includes bilateral weight-bearing anteroposterior (AP) and lateral views of the foot and ankle. Bilateral radiographs allow comparisons in patients who have unilateral disease and can be used to help explain the problem and the planned surgery to the patients.[40] Possible coexisting degenerative changes or deformities in the adjacent joints and the longitudinal arch of the foot should be identified and assessed. Different angular and linear methods of radiographic measurements can be used to quantify the degree of flatfoot deformity.[1,40–44] We routinely measure the following on the lateral weight-bearing radiographs of the ankle: lateral talus–first metatarsal angle, AP talus–first metatarsal angle, and calcaneal pitch angle and on the AP radiograph of the foot the following: AP TN coverage angle and AP talus–first metatarsal angle. Measurement of the lateral talar–first metatarsal angle using the weight-bearing lateral view of the foot/ankle was found to be accurate and the most discriminating radiographic parameter in patients with symptomatic flatfoot deformity.[42] Also, the sag sign at the NC joint should be evaluated. The break of the medial column should be measured and classified according to the anatomic system introduced by Jack.[20] Another exact and reliable radiographic method to characterize the medial longitudinal arch is the navicular height to foot length ratio.[45] On the AP view of the foot, the talar head uncoverage angle is the most important radiographic measure to quantify the flatfoot deformity.[42] For standardized assessment of varus and valgus deformity of the hindfoot, we use the Saltzman view.[46] In patients with painful osteoarthritis of the adjacent joints, single-photon emission computed tomography/computed tomography can be performed for a more accurate assessment of degenerative changes and their biologic activity.[47] Because careful clinical examination is usually sufficient to assess the PTTD, magnetic resonance imaging (MRI) is not routinely performed. However, in some cases, MRI may be helpful to evaluate the amount and localization of posterior tibial tendon and the spring ligament complex pathology and to assess the muscular atrophy.[43,48]

SURGICAL TECHNIQUE

The procedure can be performed under general or regional anesthesia. The patient is placed in a supine position. The ipsilateral back of the patient is lifted until a strictly upward position of the lower extremity is obtained. A pneumatic tourniquet is applied on the ipsilateral thigh.

A modification of the medial approach described by Knupp and colleagues[49] and De Wachter and colleagues[50] is used. A skin incision is made from the medial cuneiform toward the medial malleolus. The incision is localized parallel to the posterior tibial tendon (approximately 5 mm above the tendon). The posterior tibial tendon is exposed and opened through a horizontal incision of tendon sheath. The tendon is carefully examined. If the tendon shows degenerative changes, a debridement of the tendon is performed. Afterward, arthrotomy of the ST joint is done by a horizontal incision along the upper border of the posterior tibial tendon, paying attention not to open the capsule of the TN joint distally and not to damage the tibiocalcaneal fibers of the deltoid ligament proximally. Kirschner (K) wires are inserted into the talar neck and the sustentaculum tali, and a special distractor (Hintermann distractor; Newdeal-Integra LifeSciences, Plainsboro, NJ, USA) is mounted to open the talocalcaneal joint (**Fig. 2**A). The interosseous ligament is dissected, allowing further distraction of the ST joint. Thereafter, the talar and calcaneal surfaces are debrided to the subchondral bone. Sclerotic bony area may be fractured with a 2-mm drill bit. In the presence of major bony defects, autologous bone grafts may be considered. The distractor and the K wires are removed.

K wires are then inserted into the navicular and first cuneiform bones, and the distractor is mounted again. A small Hohmann retractor is placed dorsally onto the cuneiform to protect the anterior tibial tendon. Arthrotomy of the NC joint is completed by

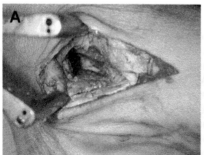
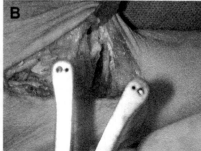

Fig. 2. Surgical exposure after debriding the joint surfaces to the subchondral bone. (*A*) ST joint. (*B*) NC joint.

sharp dissection of the medial and plantar capsule. The dorsal capsulotomy is done while stepwise increasing the distraction, allowing full visualization of all 3 NC joints (see **Fig. 2**B). Debridement of the NC joint surface is performed in a manner similar to that of the ST joint.

With the foot held in a strictly plantigrade position, the ST joint is reduced by pushing the talar head upwards laterally on the anterior aspect of the calcaneus. Two K-wires are then used to secure the preliminary fixation, the first from the tuber of the calcaneus through the posterior facet of the ST joint into the posterior aspect of the talar body and the second from the anterior process of the calcaneus into the talar head. The achieved correction of the deformity is carefully evaluated clinically and by using fluoroscopy. If the heel cannot be corrected to neutral alignment, the posterior K wire is removed and a medial displacement osteotomy of the calcaneus is performed through an additional lateral approach as described in detail by Stufkens and colleagues.[51] After the oblique osteotomy is made approximately 1 cm posterior to the peroneal tendons, the tuber fragment is mobilized and shifted medially until neutral hindfoot alignment is achieved. The posterior K wire is inserted again. At least two 7.5-mm cannulated compression screws (Qwix; Newdeal-Integra LifeSciences, Plainsboro, NJ, USA) are used to achieve rotational stability.

For reduction of the NC joint, the K wires left in the navicular and cuneiform are used as "joysticks" to enforce plantarward shifting of the cuneiform bones. Also, manipulation of the Hintermann distractor without tension helps to achieve the desired plantigrade position of the forefoot (**Fig. 3**). First, a K wire is inserted distally through the first cuneiform into the lateral aspect of navicular bone (**Fig. 4**A). The second K wire is placed from the tuberosity of the navicular bone into the second cuneiform. After the position of the K wires is checked by fluoroscopy, two 5.5-mm cannulated screws

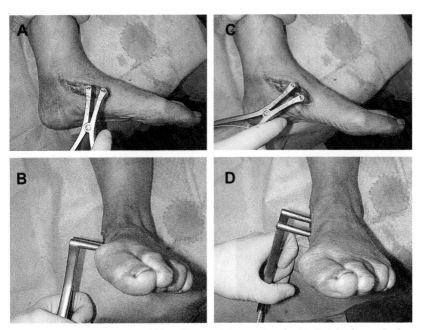

Fig. 3. Intraoperative correction of forefoot supinatus using the K wires in the navicular and first cuneiform as "joysticks" (see text). (*A, B*) Noncorrected position. (*C, D*) Corrected position.

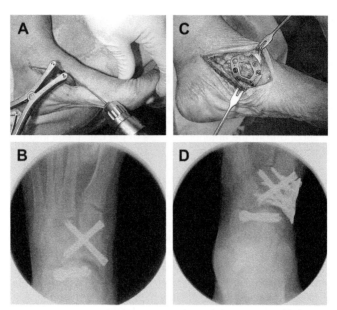

Fig. 4. Internal fixation of NC joint. (*A*) With the foot held in the corrected position, a K wire is inserted distally through the first cuneiform to the lateral aspect of navicular bone, followed by a second K wire (see text). (*B*) AP fluoroscopic view after insertion of a 5.5-mm cannulated screw. (*C*) The NC fusion is further stabilized by a medioplantar plate contributing a tension banding effect. (*D*) AP fluoroscopic view after positioning of the plate.

are inserted (see **Fig. 4**B). Third, an additional plate (Newdeal-Integra LifeSciences, Plainsboro, NJ, USA) is used at the medioplantar aspect of the midfoot to serve as a tension banding to increase the stability of NC fusion (see **Fig. 4**C, D).

The capsule of the ST joint is closed with interrupted 0 resorbable sutures. The wound is closed in layers, with the skin secured with interrupted nonabsorbable stitches. Usually, no drain is necessary. A thick compressive dressing is applied, and the foot is placed in a splint.

POSTOPERATIVE MANAGEMENT

Postoperative management in this patient cohort is identical to the aftercare in patients with double-hindfoot arthrodesis.[50] After 2 to 3 days, the compressive dressing and temporary splint are removed and replaced by a short-leg walking cast. Full weight-bearing is allowed in the cast as tolerated. At 8 weeks postoperation, the cast is removed and the bony healing of the arthrodesis is assessed via routine foot/ankle radiographs. If the bony healing occurred incompletely, the foot is further protected by a walker for another 4 to 6 weeks. If bone healing is achieved, free ambulation is permitted and a rehabilitation program, including proprioception, coordination, and strength training is initiated.

RESULTS OF TREATMENT

Combined ST and NC fusion has been performed in 10 consecutive patients (mean age 69.9 ± 6.4 [range, 58.6–80.4] years). There were 8 female and 2 male patients (10 feet; 5 right and 5 left). The mean follow-up was 1.5 ± 0.5 (range, 1.0–2.6) years.

Table 1
Radiographic assessment of postoperative angle correction in 10 patients with stage III flatfoot deformity treated with combined ST and NC fusion

Angle	Preoperative (°)	6 Mo Postoperative (°)	P Value[a]
TN Coverage	32 ± 11	19 ± 10	.02
First MT AP	16 ± 14	8 ± 12	.01
First MT Lateral	−17 ± 7	−8 ± 6	.01
Talocalcaneal	35 ± 8	30 ± 5	.04
Calcaneal Pitch	3 ± 3	5 ± 3	.02

Abbreviation: MT, metatarsal.
[a] Using Wilcoxon test.

In all 10 patients, the flatfoot deformity was significantly corrected (**Table 1**). Solid fusion at the site of arthrodesis was observed between 8 and 12 weeks (**Fig. 5**). At the latest follow-up, no loss of correction was observed clinically and radiologically, except in 1 patient. All patients were satisfied with the results of this procedure and stated that they would undergo the surgery again. All patients were able to wear normal shoes without insoles.

DISCUSSION

Numerous surgical treatment options for the correction of PTTD stage III adult flatfoot deformity have been presented and discussed.[1–5,15,38,39,43,52–55] In the 1980s, PTTD was recognized as a common cause of adult acquired flatfoot deformity.[56] Optimal management of this disease requires careful assessment and an understanding of the complex difficult-to-define biomechanics and pathophysiology.[7] In this article, we reviewed the historical perspective and current use of medial column procedures in patients with flatfoot deformity. Furthermore, we described our surgical technique, combined ST and NC fusion for extended breakdown of the medial arch in patients

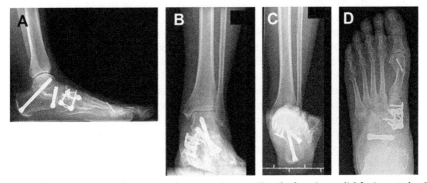

Fig. 5. Follow-up control after 1 year (same patient as **Fig. 1**), showing solid fusion at the ST and NC fusion sites. (*A*) Lateral view of the foot showing restored arch with regular reduction of the TN and TMT joints. (*B*) AP view of the ankle shows a well-balanced ankle joint complex. (*C*) The Saltzman view shows a suboptimal correction of the heel valgus. (*D*) The AP view of the foot shows a well-aligned medial column with restored talus–first metatarsal angle and physiologic navicular coverage of talar head.

with stage III acquired flatfoot deformity. Also, the preliminary results of 10 patients who underwent this procedure were presented.

Our concept was successful in this small patient cohort of 10 consecutive patients. Our results show that fusion at 2 levels, the ST and NC joints, was effective to achieve a solid correction of the flatfoot deformity in all 3 planes. After 1 year, all patients were highly satisfied with the procedure and stated that they would pursue the same treatment again. In particular, patients reported a significant improvement in proprioception and the feeling of their feet on the ground during walking and standing.

One question regarding this procedure is to what extent ST and NC fusion would be effective in correcting a subluxation of the TN joint, often observed in this patient cohort. Most surprisingly, the TN joint and the abduction deformity of the forefoot were found to be most effectively corrected by this surgical technique (see **Fig. 5**). This technique may be explained first by meticulous reduction of the talocalcaneal angle. Correction of the talocalcaneal angle, that is the physiologic position of talar head in relation to anterior surface of calcaneus (CC joint), leads to restoration of the Chopart joint. Second, the reduction and fusion of the NC joint by plantar flexion and adduction restores the biomechanics of the first ray. We believe this avoids pathologic restraints at the TN joint, explaining the success of our procedure to reduce the TN joint.

In our patient cohort, one failure occurred. In this patient, the talar head shifted medially into a plantar-flexed position. Analysis of this case showed that the preoperative severe valgus deformity of the heel was not fully corrected. The remaining valgus of the heel caused eccentric heel pull during gait, recreating pathologically increased pronation forces which were transmitted from hindfoot to midfoot. In addition, positioning of the anterior screw to fix the ST joint was not correct, which resulted in insufficient stability of the talar head against aforementioned pronation forces.

From this failure, we concluded that in addition to complete correction of valgus misalignment, rigid fixation of the ST joint is crucial for success. Thus, we advocate that at least 2 screws are used to obtain sufficient solid stability against pronation forces. Pronation forces tend to shift the talar head medially and plantarward, causing a potential failure of reduction at the TN side. The primary biomechanical stability of the fusion on the ST side is therefore one of the most important steps of the surgical procedure and should be carefully considered. In critical cases, such as in obese patients or patients with reduced bone quality, we consider use of a third screw to enhance the stability.

We did not encounter any complications at the site of NC joint fusion (eg, nonunion and loss of reduction). Obviously, selected internal fixation of the NC joint using cannulated 5.5-mm screws and a medioplantar plate was strong enough to withstand the bending forces during the gait. The inclusion of all 3 NC joints into arthrodesis may have increased the contact area and additionally supported the fusion process. Meticulous correction of valgus heel deformities and biomechanically solid fixation of the ST joint may have normalized the biomechanics and joint loads of the hindfoot, protecting the midfoot against pronation forces acting from the hindfoot and supination forces acting from the forefoot. This protection may explain the midterm stability of this corrective procedure.

SUMMARY

Combined ST and NC fusion was successful in restoring the longitudinal medial arch after extended breakdown while preserving the TN joint. This surgical technique was shown to give a reliable fusion and biomechanically stable position of the foot.

Although not exactly quantified, we strongly believe that motion at the Chopart joint, which is preserved because of limited fusion in contrast to triple fusion, may be beneficial at long term because it allows better contact force adaptation during gait. The more physiologic absorption and transfer of forces during walking and standing may also preserve the TMT joints from consecutive overloading and development of degenerative changes and destabilization.

ACKNOWLEDGMENTS

The authors wish to thank Ashley L. Kapron, BS for helpful discussion and correction of the article.

REFERENCES

1. Kelly IP, Easley ME. Treatment of stage 3 adult acquired flatfoot. Foot Ankle Clin 2001;6:153–66.
2. Myerson MS. Adult acquired flatfoot deformity: treatment of dysfunction of the posterior tibial tendon. Instr Course Lect 1997;46:393–405.
3. Francisco R, Chiodo CP, Wilson MG. Management of the rigid adult acquired flatfoot deformity. Foot Ankle Clin 2007;12:317–27.
4. Kadakia AR, Haddad SL. Hindfoot arthrodesis for the adult acquired flat foot. Foot Ankle Clin 2003;8:569–94.
5. Sizensky JA, Marks RM. Medial-sided bony procedures: why, what, and how? Foot Ankle Clin 2003;8:539–62.
6. Sangeorzan BJ, Smith D, Veith R, et al. Triple arthrodesis using internal fixation in treatment of adult foot disorders. Clin Orthop Relat Res 1993;294:299–307.
7. Van Boerum DH, Sangeorzan BJ. Biomechanics and pathophysiology of flat foot. Foot Ankle Clin 2003;8:419–30.
8. Angus PD, Cowell HR. Triple arthrodesis. A critical long-term review. J Bone Joint Surg Br 1986;68:260–5.
9. Haritidis JH, Kirkos JM, Provellegios SM, et al. Long-term results of triple arthrodesis: 42 cases followed for 25 years. Foot Ankle Int 1994;15:548–51.
10. Smith RW, Shen W, Dewitt S, et al. Triple arthrodesis in adults with non-paralytic disease. A minimum ten-year follow-up study. J Bone Joint Surg Am 2004;86:2707–13.
11. Saltzman CL, Fehrle MJ, Cooper RR, et al. Triple arthrodesis: twenty-five and forty-four-year average follow-up of the same patients. J Bone Joint Surg Am 1999;81:1391–402.
12. Kitaoka HB, Patzer GL. Subtalar arthrodesis for posterior tibial tendon dysfunction and pes planus. Clin Orthop Relat Res 1997;345:187–94.
13. Mann RA, Beaman DN, Horton GA. Isolated subtalar arthrodesis. Foot Ankle Int 1998;19:511–9.
14. Stephens HM, Walling AK, Solmen JD, et al. Subtalar repositional arthrodesis for adult acquired flatfoot. Clin Orthop Relat Res 1999;365:69–73.
15. Cohen BE, Johnson JE. Subtalar arthrodesis for treatment of posterior tibial tendon insufficiency. Foot Ankle Clin 2001;6:121–8.
16. Miller OL. A plastic flat foot operation. J Bone Joint Surg Am 1927;9:84–91.
17. Fraser RK, Menelaus MB, Williams PF, et al. The Miller procedure for mobile flat feet. J Bone Joint Surg Br 1995;77:396–9.
18. Hoke M. An operation for the correction of extremely relaxed flat feet. J Bone Joint Surg Am 1931;13:773–83.

19. Butte FL. Navicular-cuneiform arthrodesis for flat-foot: an end-result study. J Bone Joint Surg Am 1937;19:496–502.
20. Jack EA. Naviculo-cuneiform fusion in the treatment of flat foot. J Bone Joint Surg Br 1953;35:82.
21. Seymour N. The late results of naviculo-cuneiform fusion. J Bone Joint Surg Br 1967;49:558–9.
22. Duncan JW, Lovell WW. Modified Hoke-Miller flatfoot procedure. Clin Orthop Relat Res 1983;181:24–7.
23. Caldwell GD. Surgical correction of relaxed flatfoot by the Durham flatfoot plasty. Clin Orthop Relat Res 1953;2:221–6.
24. Greisberg J, Assal M, Hansen ST Jr, et al. Isolated medial column stabilization improves alignment in adult-acquired flatfoot. Clin Orthop Relat Res 2005;435:197–202.
25. Chi TD, Toolan BC, Sangeorzan BJ, et al. The lateral column lengthening and medial column stabilization procedures. Clin Orthop Relat Res 1999;365:81–90.
26. Coetzee JC, Hansen ST. Surgical management of severe deformity resulting from posterior tibial tendon dysfunction. Foot Ankle Int 2001;22:944–9.
27. Fortin PT. Posterior tibial tendon insufficiency. Isolated fusion of the talonavicular joint. Foot Ankle Clin 2001;6:137–51.
28. O'Malley MJ, Deland JT, Lee KT. Selective hindfoot arthrodesis for the treatment of adult acquired flatfoot deformity: an in vitro study. Foot Ankle Int 1995;16:411–7.
29. Astion DJ, Deland JT, Otis JC, et al. Motion of the hindfoot after simulated arthrodesis. J Bone Joint Surg Am 1997;79:241–6.
30. Fishco WD, Cornwall MW. Gait analysis after talonavicular joint fusion: 2 case reports. J Foot Ankle Surg 2004;43:241–7.
31. Fogel GR, Katoh Y, Rand JA, et al. Talonavicular arthrodesis for isolated arthrosis: 9.5-year results and gait analysis. Foot Ankle 1982;3:105–13.
32. Harper MC, Tisdel CL. Talonavicular arthrodesis for the painful adult acquired flatfoot. Foot Ankle Int 1996;17:658–61.
33. Harper MC. Talonavicular arthrodesis for the acquired flatfoot in the adult. Clin Orthop Relat Res 1999;365:65–8.
34. Camasta CA, Menke CR, Hall PB. A review of 51 talonavicular joint arthrodeses for flexible pes valgus deformity. J Foot Ankle Surg 2010;49:113–8.
35. Easley ME, Trnka HJ, Schon LC, et al. Isolated subtalar arthrodesis. J Bone Joint Surg Am 2000;82:613–24.
36. Chahal J, Stephen DJ, Bulmer B, et al. Factors associated with outcome after subtalar arthrodesis. J Orthop Trauma 2006;20:555–61.
37. Hintermann B, Gachter A. The first metatarsal rise sign: a simple, sensitive sign of tibialis posterior tendon dysfunction. Foot Ankle Int 1996;17:236–41.
38. Churchill RS, Sferra JJ. Posterior tibial tendon insufficiency. Its diagnosis, management, and treatment. Am J Orthop 1998;27:339–47.
39. Johnson KA, Strom DE. Tibialis posterior tendon dysfunction. Clin Orthop Relat Res 1989;239:196–206.
40. Beals TC, Pomeroy GC, Manoli A. Posterior tibial tendon insufficiency: diagnosis and treatment. J Am Acad Orthop Surg 1999;7:112–8.
41. Chadha H, Pomeroy G, Manoli A. Radiologic signs of unilateral pes planus. Foot Ankle Int 1997;18:603–4.
42. Younger AS, Sawatzky B, Dryden P. Radiographic assessment of adult flatfoot. Foot Ankle Int 2005;26:820–5.

43. Giza E, Cush G, Schon LC. The flexible flatfoot in the adult. Foot Ankle Clin 2007; 12:251–71.
44. Pomeroy GC, Pike RH, Beals TC, et al. Acquired flatfoot in adults due to dysfunction of the posterior tibial tendon. J Bone Joint Surg Am 1999;81:1173–82.
45. Saltzman CL, Nawoczenski DA, Talbot KD. Measurement of the medial longitudinal arch. Arch Phys Med Rehabil 1995;76:45–9.
46. Saltzman CL, el Khoury GY. The hindfoot alignment view. Foot Ankle Int 1995;16: 572–6.
47. Pagenstert GI, Barg A, Leumann AG, et al. SPECT-CT imaging in degenerative joint disease of the foot and ankle. J Bone Joint Surg Br 2009;91:1191–6.
48. Wacker J, Calder JD, Engstrom CM, et al. MR morphometry of posterior tibialis muscle in adult acquired flat foot. Foot Ankle Int 2003;24:354–7.
49. Knupp M, Schuh R, Stufkens SA, et al. Subtalar and talonavicular arthrodesis through a single medial approach for the correction of severe planovalgus deformity. J Bone Joint Surg Br 2009;91:612–5.
50. De Wachter J, Knupp M, Hintermann B. Double-hindfoot arthrodesis through a single medial approach. Tech Foot Ankle Surg 2007;6:237–42.
51. Stufkens SA, Knupp M, Hintermann B. Medial displacement calcaneal osteotomy. Tech Foot Ankle Surg 2009;8:85–90.
52. Pinney SJ, Van Bergeyk A. Controversies in surgical reconstruction of acquired adult flat foot deformity. Foot Ankle Clin 2003;8:595–604.
53. McCormack AP, Ching RP, Sangeorzan BJ. Biomechanics of procedures used in adult flatfoot deformity. Foot Ankle Clin 2001;6:15–23.
54. Neufeld SK, Myerson MS. Complications of surgical treatments for adult flatfoot deformities. Foot Ankle Clin 2001;6:179–91.
55. Coetzee JC, Castro MD. The indications and biomechanical rationale for various hindfoot procedures in the treatment of posterior tibialis tendon dysfunction. Foot Ankle Clin 2003;8:453–9.
56. Funk DA, Cass JR, Johnson KA. Acquired adult flat foot secondary to posterior tibial-tendon pathology. J Bone Joint Surg Am 1986;68:95–102.

Arthroscopic Arthodesis of Subtalar Joint

Gerardo Muñoz Muraro, MD, PhD[a],*,
Patricio Fuentes Carvajal, MD[b]

KEYWORDS

• Arthroscopic • Subtalar • Arthrodesis • Pain • Hindfoot • Joint

Isolated subtalar arthrodesis is well accepted for treatment of pathologic conditions of the subtalar joint associated with pain, instability, and deformity that do not respond to conservative treatment. The most frequent indications are primary talocalcaneal or posttraumatic arthrosis (talus or calcaneal fracture); congenital malformations (coalition); or inflammatory diseases.[1]

Isolated subtalar arthrodesis is superior to double or triple arthrodesis, such as to preserve some hindfoot mobility, thereby being of smaller risk for secondary degenerative disease of neighboring joints and nonunion or malunion of the tarsal transversal joint.[2] The amount of mobility loss on performing the isolated subtalar arthrodesis is less than a double or triple arthrodesis. It is known that the function of the talonavicular joint has the greatest influence on overall hindfoot function.[3]

The published results of the open techniques are satisfactory, with a range of union between 84% and 95% and with few complications, such as symptomatic hardware protrusion (20%), infection (3%), hindfoot misalignment (6%), lateral impingement (10%), and sural nerve injury (9%).[1,2]

ARTHROSCOPIC SUBTALAR ARTHRODESIS

The development of arthroscopic surgery gives the surgeon a valuable alternative to perform subtalar arthrodesis that results in faster recovery, less pain, and fewer perioperative complications. The procedure was first developed in 1992 by Tasto[4] and later presented at the Arthroscopy Association of North America's Annual meeting in 1994. In 2003, the same author reported bony union after 8 to 9 weeks in all 25

The authors have nothing to disclosure.
[a] Departamento de Traumatología, Clínica Las Condes, Lo Fontecilla 441, Las Condes, Santiago, Chile
[b] Clínica Santa María, Avenida Santa Maria 0500, Providencia, Santiago, Chile
* Corresponding author.
E-mail address: gmunoz@clc.cl

Foot Ankle Clin N Am 16 (2011) 83–90
doi:10.1016/j.fcl.2010.12.007
1083-7515/11/$ – see front matter © 2011 Elsevier Inc. All rights reserved.

patients.[5] Thereafter, many surgeons have reported this technique using different portals.[6–22]

Indications and Contraindications

Isolated arthrodesis of the subtalar joint has been proposed for the treatment of primary arthrosis, posttraumatic arthrosis, rheumatoid arthritis, and talocalcaneal coalition. Previous calcaneal and talar fractures are the most common conditions for development of posttraumatic osteoarthritis.[7,8]

Theoretically, the advantage of the arthroscopic subtalar arthrodesis is to preserve talar and calcaneal blood supply and the surrounding soft tissues from further damages, which may be of particular importance after previous traumas and surgeries. Further, it may preserve foot propioception. The perioperative morbidity was supposed to be inferior to that with open techniques.[6,7] These advantages become more important in patients with high-risk factors who may develop soft tissue complications, such as patients with diabetes or peripheral vascular alterations, and smokers.

Relative contraindications for arthroscopic subtalar arthrodesis are single and multiplane deformities. However, the limitations of deformities are not yet defined in the literature. In malunion, open technique might be mandatory to correct the deformity.[9] Other contraindications for arthroscopic subtalar arthrodesis are previous failed arthrodesis because of arthrofibrosis and local scar, where a wider approach and extended debridement are required.[10] The necessity to perform a concomitant midfoot or forefoot procedure is also a contraindication when the arthroscopic approach is performed through posterior portals in the prone position.[7,11,12]

There are some controversies with regard to posttraumatic arthrosis after calcaneal fracture. Joint narrowing and subtalar arthrofibrosis were suggested to be a contraindication by some authors,[4,13] whereas others do not see a contraindication as long as there is no joint collapse or loss of stock bone.[15]

Surgical Technique

The procedure is performed under general or regional anesthesia. The patient position depends on the portals to be used. It can be supine, lateral, or prone position. A tourniquet is used to obtain better joint visualization. It may be opened to verify a bleeding surface before internal fixation of the subtalar joint.[7,10,14] The use of soft tissue traction may facilitate joint visualization. The use of bone traction is not described as an alternative for the arthroscopic subtalar arthrodesis.[7,10–12,15]

The classic portals for the subtalar arthroscopy are the anterolateral and posterolateral. Besides these, additional portals may be used for further visualization, joint distraction, and instrumentation.[15,16] The use of fluoroscopy may be helpful to identify the portals (**Fig. 1**).[14]

El Shazly and colleagues[15] performed arthroscopy arthrodesis through anterolateral and posterolateral portals. They also described an accessory anterolateral portal for subtalar instrumentation and visualization, 1-cm distal and 0.5-cm anterior to the tip of the lateral maleolus (**Fig. 2**).

In 2000, Van Dijk and coworkers[17] described the use of posteriors portals for subtalar and ankle arthroscopy. The posterolateral is done immediately laterally to the Achilles tendon. The posteromedial portal is then used to insert the instruments while using the posterolateral portal and the flexor hallucis longus tendon as a reference. The author suggested that posterior portals allow a better visualization of the posterior subtalar facet. Lee and colleagues[7] also reported this procedure in 16 patients using only posterolateral and posteromedial portals (**Fig. 3**).

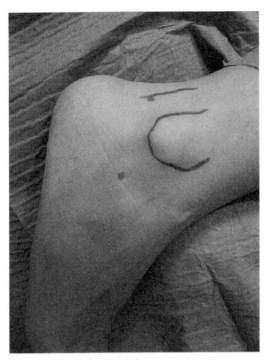

Fig. 1. Anterolateral and posterolateral portals.

Sitler and colleagues,[18] in a cadaveric study, found a distance of 6.4 mm from the posteromedial portal to the tibial nerve, a distance of 9.6 mm to the posterior tibial artery, and a distance of 17.1 mm to calcaneal branch of the tibial nerve. This shows that there is enough secure space to perform the posterior arthroscopy.

Beimers and colleagues[8] described arthroscopic subtalar arthrodesis in patients with talocalcaneal coalition using posterior portals. They added a third accessory portal through the sinus tarsi, which permits a safe joint distraction and

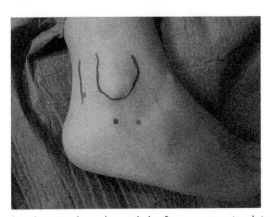

Fig. 2. Anterolateral and posterolateral portals (*red*); accesory anterolateral portal (*green*).

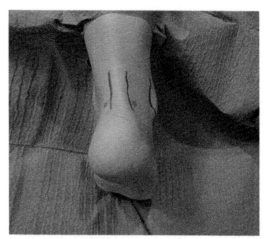

Fig. 3. Posterolateral and posteromedial portals.

instrumentation of the anterior portion of posterior facet. Similarly, Lee and colleagues[10] and Amendola and colleagues[11] described the procedure through posterior approaches, adding a third portal, placed 1-cm proximal and 1-cm posterior to the tip of the maleolus, which is used for joint distraction (**Fig. 4**).

Both arthroscopic approaches for subtalar arthrodesis have a high success rate and few complications. The choosing of one or the other, in general, depends on the surgeon's experience and the specific requirements of each patient.

Optics of 2.7, 2.9, or 4 mm can be used, and they can be indistinctly used in the different portals. The visualization and instrumentation is easer with smaller optics as typically 2.7 and 2.9 mm in diameter.[12] The resection of joint cartilage is performed with different instruments, such as curettes, chisels, drill, and shaver.

It is widely accepted that it is only necessary to debride the posterior facet to obtain subtalar fusion. However, it could be that this is mainly because of the difficulty encountered in accessing the middle and anterior facets through the posterior

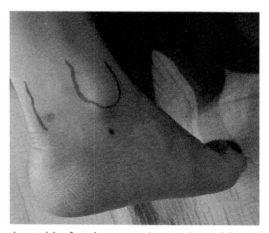

Fig. 4. Posterolateral portal (*red*) and accesory sinus tarsi portal (*green*).

arthroscopy portals.[6,19] Nevertheless, it should be kept in mind that in some instances, such as a big middle-anterior subtalar coalition without posterior involvement, a complete subtalar fusion may be required to resolve the problem, as reported by some authors[14]

The advantage of preserving the interosseous ligament is to preserve the bone blood supply, which may decrease the vascular necrosis risk or the fusion from slowing. However, most open techniques resect the interosseus ligament through a sinus tarsi approach, and they do not report larger fusion times or avascular necrosis, so that it is only a theoretical advantage.

Intraoperative fluoroscopy can be useful to check the extent of joint debridement in the case of difficult arthroscopic visualization. In general, joint debridement of 1 to 2 mm of subchondral bone is required for getting a bleeding bony surface, which in turn may be ideal for obtaining primary bony healing. Adding a bone graft can facilitate this process, as reported by several authors.[10,14,20] Flemister and colleagues[20] recommended the use of bone graft routinely in subtalar arthrodesis. Glanzman and Sanhueza-Hernandez[14] used tricortical and cancellous bone graft through the posterolateral portal routinely. Lee and colleagues[10] reported the use of autograft through the posterolateral portal by means of a funnel.

El Shazly and colleagues,[15] in contrast, reported a 100% fusion rate (10 patients) without the use of any bone graft. Lee and colleagues[7] most recently reported in 16 patients who underwent an arthrodesis through posterior portals without bone graft a union rate of 94%.

The arthrodesis fixation is obtained with talocalcaneal screws. One or two screws are generally used. The arthroscopic technique may allow the surgeon to control the position of the screws during insertion. Prone position of the patient may facilitate the screw insertion.[7]

El Shazly and colleagues[15] reported a 100% fusion rate with one cannulated 7-mm screw from talus to calcaneus. Lee and coworkers[7,10] used two cannulated 6.5- or 7.3-mm screws from calcaneus to talus. Amendola and colleagues[11] used two cannulated 6.5-mm screws in 10 patients. Glanzmann and Sanhueza-Hernandez[14] used one cannulated 7- or 7.5-mm screw. There was no difference found between one or two screw fixation techniques with regard to obtained healing. However, no study provided accurate information about changes of position at fusion site.

RESULTS

Surgical time for arthroscopic subtalar arthrodesis varied between 58 and 90 minutes.[7,8,14,21] It was generally longer in the beginning, indicating that there is a short learning curve.

One of the advantages of the arthroscopic procedure may be the hospitalization period. Scranton[22] reported an average decrease of 1.7 hospitalization days using the arthroscopic technique. Glanzmann and Sanhueza-Hernandez[14] report an average hospitalization time of 2 days. The return to daily activities after arthroscopic technique was 16 weeks after surgery[6] and the average work reincorporation was 27 weeks.[14]

Easly and colleagues[1] reported a union rate of 84% in 148 patients after open surgical techniques. This was inferior to the reported results using arthroscopic techniques with a healing rate of 97% (range, 91%–100%) and a healing time of 11.2 weeks (8.9–15 weeks) (**Table 1**).[7,8,11,14,15,21,22]

Scranton[22] compared 17 in situ subtalar arthrodesis patients with open technique (12 patients) with arthroscopic arthrodesis (five patients). At follow-up, a fusion was

Table 1
Arthroscopic techniques

Author	N	Preoperative Diagnosis	Technique (portals)	Fusion Rate (%)	Average Time of Fusion (weeks)	AOFAS
Scranton[22] (1999)	5	Subtalar arthrosis	AL, PL, PLacc	100	n/r	n/r
Tasto[4,5] (2003)	25	Subtalar arthrosis	AL, PL	100	8,9	n/r
Glanzmann and Sanhueza-Hernandez[14] (2007)	41	Primary arthritis, posttraumatic osteoarthritis	AL, PL	100	11	53–84
Amendola et al[11] (2007)	11	Primary arthritis, posttraumatic osteoarthritis, tarsal coalition	PL, PLacc, PM	91	10	36–86
Beimers et al[8] (2009)	3	Tarsal coalition	PL, PM, PLacc	100	6	n/r
El Shazly et al[15] (2009)	10	Posttraumatic arthritis (calcaneal fracture)	AL, ALacc, PL	100	11.4	38–74
Gómez et al[21] (2010)	12	Posttraumatic arthrosis	PL, PM, PLacc	84	15	n/r
Lee et al[7] (2010)	16	Posttraumatic arthritis (calcaneal fracture)	PL, PM	94	11	35–84

Abbreviations: AL, anterolateral; ALacc, accesory anterolateral; AOFAS, American Orthopaedic Foot & Ankle Society score; PL, posterolateral; PLacc, accesory postrolateral; PM, posteromedial.

found in all five patients after arthroscopy and in 11 of the 12 patients after an open technique.

In general the isolated subtalar arthrodesis gains good functional results and with a high patient satisfaction. This is also documented for arthroscopic subtalar arthrodesis with overall excellent results and improvement in functional score.

Risk factors for nonunion after open subtalar arhrodesis are smoking, more than 2 mm avascular bone, and failed previous arthrodesis.[1] Other factors related to bad results are peroneal tendon impingement, sural nerve lesion, and fat pad atrophy.[12]

Complications after open arthrodesis were reported to be as high as 5% to 16% for nonunion, 3% to 30% for superficial infections, 2.5% to 5% for deep infections, 6% for symptomatic misalignment, 20% for hardware irritation, 12% for hardware failure, and 2% for complex regional pain syndrome.[12]

With the use of arthroscopic subtalar arthrodesis, by contrast, fewer complications were found. For instance, in the series by Lee and coworkers,[7] of 16 patients there was only one deep infection related to screw failure and nonunion in the same patient. Other complications were chronic ankle pain, peroneal tendonitis, and pseudoarthrosis.[7,11,14,21]

SUMMARY

Although the use of arthroscopy was found to be a safe technique with a small complication rate, the results of the rather small patient series must be considered with caution when comparing with open techniques. First, they may have included selected patient with no or very little deformity, which are the ideal conditions for successful isolated subtalar fusion. Second, no study has used CT scan to assess bone healing at the fusion site. Third, fixation technique was not done in a standardized manner.

It must be emphasized that the main limitation to the use of arthroscopic techniques is the absence of any deformity. The main goal for every subtalar fusion is to obtain a subtalar fusion in a correct position of talus with regard to the calcaneus and navicular bone. If this cannot be achieved by arthroscopic techniques, an open procedure should be chosen.

REFERENCES

1. Easley ME, Trnka HJ, Schon LC, et al. Isolated subtalar arthrodesis. J Bone Joint Surg Am 2000;82(5):613–24.
2. Mann RA, Beaman DN, Horton GA. Isolated subtalar arthrodesis. Foot Ankle Int 1998;19:511–9.
3. Savory K, Wülker N, Stukenborg C, et al. Biomechanics of the hindfoot joints in response to degenerative hindfoot arthrodeses. Clin Biomech 1998;13:62–70.
4. Tasto JP. Subtalar arthroscopy. In: Mcginty JB, Burkhart SS, Jackson RW, et al, editors. Operative arthroscopy. 3rd edition. New York: Lippincott Williams & Wilkins; 2003. p. 944–52.
5. Tasto JP. Arthroscopic subtalar arthrodesis. Tech Foot Ankle Surg 2003;2:122–8.
6. Frey C. Surgical advancements: arthroscopic alternatives to open procedures: great toe, subtalar joint, Haglund's deformity, and tendoscopy. Foot Ankle Clin N Am 2009;14:313–39.
7. Lee K, Park CH, Seon JK, et al. Arthroscopic subtalar arthrodesis using a posterior 2-portal approach in the prone position. Arthroscopy 2010;26(2):230–8.
8. Beimers L, De Leeuw P, Van Dijk N. A 3-portal approach for arthroscopic subtalar artrodesis. Knee Surg Sports Traumatol Arthrosc 2009;17:830–4.

9. Radnay C, Clare M, Sanders R. Subtalar fusion after displaced intra-articular calcaneal fractures: does initial operative treatment matter? J Bone Joint Surg Am 2010;92(Suppl 1, Pt 1):32–43.
10. Lee KB, Saltzman CL, Suh JS, et al. A posterior 3-portal arthroscopic approach for isolated subtalar arthrodesis. Arthroscopy 2008;24(11):1306–10.
11. Amendola A, Lee KB, Saltzman CL, et al. Technique and early experience with posterior arthroscopic subtalar arthrodesis. Foot Ankle Int 2007;28(3):298–302.
12. Robinson J, Murphy A. Arthrodesis as salvage for calcaneal malunions. Foot Ankle Clin N Am 2002;7:107–20.
13. Ferkel RD. Subtalar arthroscopy. In: Ferkle RD, Whipple TL, editors. Arthroscopic surgery: the foot and ankle. Philadelphia: Lippincott-Raven; 1996. p. 231–54.
14. Glanzmann M, Sanhueza-Hernandez R. Arthroscopic subtalar arthrodesis for symptomatic osteoarthritis of the hindfoot: a prospective study of 41 cases. Foot Ankle Int 2007;28(1):2–7.
15. El Shazly O, Nassar W, El Badrawy A. Arthroscopic subtalar fusion for post-traumatic subtalar arthritis. Arthroscopy 2009;25(7):783–7.
16. Beimers H, Frey C, van Dijk N. Arthroscopy of the posterior subtalar joint. Foot Ankle 2006;11:369–90.
17. van Dijk CN, Scholten PE, Krips R. A 2-portal endoscopic approach for diagnosis and treatment of posterior ankle pathology. Arthroscopy 2000;16:871–6.
18. Sitler DF, Amendola A, Bailey CS, et al. Posterior ankle arthroscopy: an anatomic study. J Bone Joint Surg Am 2002;84:763–9.
19. Stroud C. Arthroscopic arthrodesis of the ankle, subtalar, and first metatarsophalangeal joint. Foot Ankle Clin N Am 2002;7:135–46.
20. Flemister AS Jr, Infante AF, Sanders RW, et al. Subtalar arthrodesis for complications of intraarticular calcaneal fractures. Foot Ankle Int 2000;21(5):392–9.
21. Gómez J, Musatadi M, Martínez J. Artrodesis subastragalina artroscópica. Revista Española de Cirugía Osteoarticular 2010;45(241):1–4.
22. Scranton P. Comparison of open isolated subtalar arthrodesis with autogenous bone graft versus outpatient arthroscopic subtalar arthrodesis using injectable bone morphogenic protein-enhanced graft. Foot Ankle Int 1999;20(3):162–5.

The Anatomic Compression Arthrodesis Technique with Anterior Plate Augmentation for Ankle Arthrodesis

Michael P. Clare, MD[a],*, Roy W. Sanders, MD[b]

KEYWORDS

• Ankle arthritis • Arthrodesis • Anterior plate

Ankle arthrodesis remains the gold standard for treatment of end-stage ankle arthritis. Nonunion rates have historically been as high as 40%, largely because of destabilizing surgical techniques, such as resection of the fibula and medial malleolus, and primitive fixation techniques.[1] High rates of infection and amputation have additionally been reported.[2–4] A recent meta-analysis by Haddad and colleagues[1] reported an average nonunion rate of 10% for ankle arthrodesis using modern surgical techniques. Delayed union and nonunion of the arthrodesis result in increased patient morbidity because of prolonged immobilization and the need for secondary surgical procedures.

MODERN FIXATION TECHNIQUES

Multiple techniques have been described for ankle arthrodesis. Although various external fixation constructs have historically been used, the development of internal compression techniques through open, mini-open, and arthroscopic approaches has resulted in higher rates of union with fewer complications than external fixation.[5–7]

Holt and colleagues[6] described the anatomic compression arthrodesis technique in 1991, reporting a 93% union rate. Principles of their technique include preservation of

The authors have nothing to disclose.

[a] Division of Foot & Ankle Surgery, Florida Orthopaedic Institute, 13020 Telecom Parkway North, Tampa, FL 33637, USA
[b] Orthopaedic Trauma Service, Tampa General Hospital, Florida Orthopaedic Institute, 2 Columbia Drive, #710, Tampa, FL 33606, USA
* Corresponding author.
E-mail address: mpclare@verizon.net

bony anatomy, minimal bone resection, drilling of the subchondral plate, and rigid multiplanar screw fixation. This technique, however, features screws outside the primary plane of motion of the ankle joint, and biomechanical testing has shown that these constructs can have variable stiffness depending on the bone quality.[8–10] Patients with poor bone quality who are at risk for delayed union and nonunion may therefore require a more rigid construct. It is well-established that increasing the rigidity of an internal fixation construct decreases the incidence of delayed union and nonunion.[11]

BIOMECHANICAL RATIONALE OF THE ANTERIOR PLATE

Mears and colleagues[12] first described an anterior plate for ankle arthrodesis in 1991. They used a 4.5-mm two-hole narrow dynamic compression plate and 4.5-mm cortical screws alone as a tension band device, and theorized that the plate combined with an intact heelcord provided anterior and posterior compression forces across the ankle joint. They reported a union rate of 82% in 17 patients.

In 1995, the senior author began adding a low-profile anterior plate in selected cases as a supplement to multiplanar screws, and soon observed that arthrodesis union was more consistent and predictable. The plate was intended to be a neutralization device to provide protection for the lag effect of the multiplanar screws.

In a biomechanical model, Tarkin and colleagues[8] showed that anterior plate supplementation of multiplanar screw fixation provided increased rigidity compared with screw fixation alone. The anterior plate increased construct stiffness by a factor of 3.5 in the sagittal plane, 1.9 in the axial plane, and 1.4 in the coronal plane. Biomechanically, the anterior plate acts as a tension band, buttress, or neutralization plate when resisting plantarflexion, dorsiflexion, and torsion moments, respectively. The investigators concluded that the increased rigidity provided by the anterior plate effectively counters the forces, particularly the cantilever bending forces in the sagittal plane, which may lead to failure of a multiplanar screw construct.

Kakarala and Rajan[13] showed in a small comparative series a faster time to union with an anterior contoured plate and cross screw fixation than with cross screw fixation alone. Clare and colleagues[14] recently reported a 96% union rate in 275 ankle arthrodeses using multiplanar, partially threaded screws augmented with a nonlocking anterior plate.

Anatomically contoured, anterior locking plates have recently emerged as a fixation option for ankle arthrodesis. When placed in the absence of multiplanar screws, these implants function as tension band constructs, transforming the distraction forces of the Achilles tendon to compression forces across the ankle joint. Plaass and colleagues[15] reported a 100% union rate in 29 patients using a locked anterior double plating technique, both with and without structural bone grafting. Guo and colleagues[16] similarly reported predictable healing rates using an anatomically contoured locking plate in 10 patients, half of whom had bone defects.

STRUCTURAL GRAFT OPTIONS IN BONE LOSS

In the event of severe bone loss, structural bone graft may be required to preserve limb length and optimize the mechanical function of the surrounding joints. Depending on the dimensions of the defect and clinical scenario, structural graft options include iliac crest allograft, femoral head allograft, and iliac crest autograft. With modern fixation techniques, union rates are similar between structural allograft and structural autograft.[15,17,18] Plaass and colleagues[15] had a 100% union rate among a subset of 13 patients treated with structural allograft and locked anterior double plating. Berkowitz and colleagues[17] reported union in 10 of 11 (90.9%) failed total ankle arthroplasties treated with ankle arthrodeses using structural allograft and stabilized with multiplanar lag screws and a nonlocking anterior plate. Culpan and colleagues[18] reported union in 15 of 16 (93.7%) ankle arthrodesis using iliac crest tricortical autograft and internal fixation after failed total ankle arthroplasty.

OPERATIVE TECHNIQUE
Positioning

During the procedure, the patient is placed supine on a radiolucent table. A nonsterile bolster is placed beneath the hip and a pneumatic tourniquet is applied to the upper thigh of the operative limb. Protective padding is placed beneath the peroneal nerve and the heel of the contralateral nonoperative limb. The contralateral limb is secured to the operating table to allow rotation of the table to facilitate exposure of the anterior ankle as necessary. The ipsilateral iliac crest is prepared and draped as necessary in the event of severe bone loss.

Approach

A standard anterior approach is developed using the interval between the tibialis anterior and extensor hallucis longus tendons. Peripheral branches of the superficial peroneal nerve are identified and protected. These branches are typically found at the distal limb of the incision, at the level of the talonavicular joint. The extensor retinaculum is incised lateral to the tibialis anterior tendon while preserving the tibialis anterior tendon sheath, and the adjacent neurovascular bundle is protected. Extraperiosteal dissection is completed medially and laterally, followed by an anterior arthrotomy. A subtotal synovectomy is performed and prominent osteophytes are resected with a small osteotome.

Joint Preparation

An A/O laminar spreader is placed within the ankle joint for distraction and visualization. Meticulous joint preparation is performed using a sharp periosteal elevator and pituitary rongeur while preserving the underlying subchondral plate. The fibula is preserved in all cases. After joint irrigation, the subchondral plate is drilled with a 2.5-mm drill bit to stimulate vascular ingrowth (**Fig. 1**). In the absence of bone loss, supplemental allograft paste is placed within the ankle joint.

Assessment of Bone Loss

Erosive changes and partial joint collapse of either the tibial plafond or talar body may be identified, particularly in the event of angular deformity through the ankle joint. In this instance, the bony defect can be filled with cancellous autograft harvested from the ipsilateral proximal tibia.

The authors prefer structural bone graft in cases of severe bone loss, such as with failed total ankle arthroplasty. The height, width, and depth of the defect are measured. The residual talar body must be assessed to ensure sufficient remaining bone stock to allow rigid fixation while preserving the subtalar joint; the arthrodesis is extended to the subtalar joint in the event of inadequate bone stock. Depending on the dimensions of the defect, they typically use iliac crest allograft, which can be positioned as structural inlay graft (see later discussion), or femoral head allograft, which can be shaped to precisely match the bony defect. With structural allograft, the authors typically soak the graft segments in highly concentrated platelet aspirate to stimulate bony ingrowth.

The authors prefer iliac crest autograft in the instance of talar body osteonecrosis and failed total ankle arthroplasty that has a history of deep infection. The height, width, and depth of the defect are measured, and the height measurement is doubled.

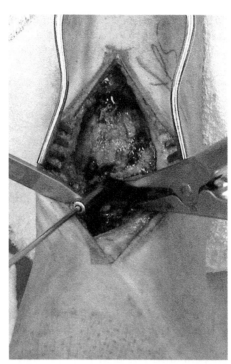

Fig. 1. Joint preparation: after cartilage removal, multiple perforations are made in the subchondral plate with a 2.5-mm drill bit to stimulate vascular ingrowth.

A tricortical trapezoidal-shaped segment is harvested to allow positioning of the graft as structural inlay graft, thereby optimizing cancellous bone apposition.[19] The inlay grafts are oriented like books on a shelf, with the width of the iliac crest resembling the binding of the book and corresponding to the width of the defect; the depth of the graft segment matches the depth of the defect; and the length of the segment should be double the height of the defect. The harvested segment in then cut at the midpoint of the length of the graft, thereby producing two autograft segments that collectively match the dimensions of the defect (**Fig. 2**).

Alternatively, the height measurement of the defect can be tripled to produce three autograft segments. The trapezoidal shape of the graft equates to more height posteriorly relative to anteriorly, thereby facilitating a neutral, plantigrade arthrodesis position. Supplemental allograft paste is placed surrounding the graft as necessary.

Joint Positioning

The ankle joint must be aligned in a neutral, plantigrade position to facilitate a heel-to-toe gait. Clare and colleagues[14] described the tibial–hindfoot axis, in which a line drawn through the center of the intramedullary canal of the tibia should be collinear to a line drawn perpendicular to the sole of the foot extending through the midportion of the talar body (lateral process) on a weight-bearing lateral radiograph (**Fig. 3**). In posttraumatic cases, particularly after pilon fractures, the talus tends to translate anteriorly with the progression of arthritic change. Contracture of the posterior capsule or Achilles tendon may also contribute to plantarflexion (equinus) malpositioning. A noncollinear tibial–hindfoot axis suggests anterior translation and plantarflexion malpositioning, both of which have the mechanical effect of lengthening the lever

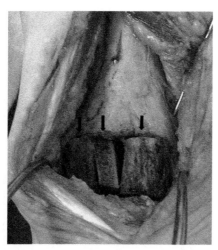

Fig. 2. Structural inlay graft: the orientation of the graft segments (*black arrows*) resembles books on a shelf, which optimizes cancellous bone apposition while maintaining limb length.

arm of the foot, making it more difficult for patients to vault over the top of the foot with gait. In most instances, a posterior capsular release, with or without a gastrocnemius recession or tendoachilles lengthening, will facilitate sufficient dorsiflexion and posterior translation of the talus to reestablish a neutral, collinear tibial–hindfoot axis. This posterior release can, however, have a deleterious effect on the tension band pull of the heel cord, counteracting the anterior plate, and may therefore decrease compression forces across the arthrodesis site. Less commonly, tapering of the posterior tibial plafond may be required.

Fixation

With the ankle joint held in neutral position, internal compression is achieved using three large partially threaded, cannulated screws in a multiplanar configuration. The first screw is placed from the metaphyseal flare of the medial distal tibia into the medial talar body, as vertically oriented as possible in both the anterior–posterior and lateral planes. A second screw is placed from the posterior malleolus along the longitudinal axis of the talar neck and into the talar head. A third screw is placed from the anterolateral distal tibia into the anterolateral talar body (**Fig. 4**). The medial and anterolateral screws are countersunk to avoid superficial prominence. Biomechanically, the initial lag screw is the only true compression screw, whereas subsequent screws act primarily as neutralization screws.

A five-hole, nonlocking small fragment reconstruction plate is then contoured; a small anterior bend is created at the distal-most screw hole to accommodate the orientation of the talar neck anteriorly. Two 3.5-mm cortical screws are first placed in the talus, followed by two similar screws placed in the distal tibia. The proximal-most screw should diverge away from the plate proximally to lessen the stress riser effect of the anterior plate (see **Fig. 4**). A locking reconstruction plate may be used in selected cases, particularly when large screw purchase is limited because of marginal bone quality. In this instance, the plate acts as a neutralization device, providing protection to the large, multiplanar screws. Alternatively, the anterior plate could be applied with a compression device before or in lieu of the large, multiplanar screws, in which case the plate would function as a true tension band device.[15]

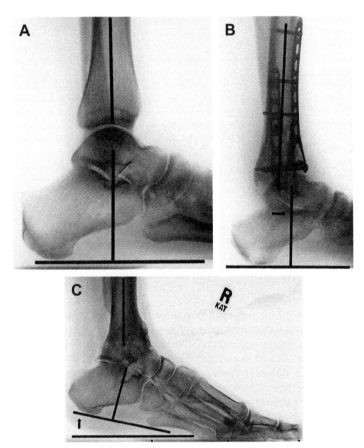

Fig. 3. Tibial–hindfoot axis. (*A*) A line drawn through the center of the intramedullary canal of the tibia should be collinear to a line drawn perpendicular to the sole of the foot extending through the midportion of the talar body (lateral process) on a weight-bearing lateral radiograph. (*B*) Noncollinear axis from anterior translation (*black arrow*): end-stage posttraumatic ankle arthritis after a pilon fracture with an unreconstructable articular surface. (*C*) Noncollinear axis from plantarflexion malalignment (*black arrow*): note also resection of the distal fibula.

Closure

The wound is irrigated and the extensor retinaculum is meticulously closed with #0 absorbable suture, followed by subcutaneous closure with 2-0 absorbable suture. The skin layer is closed with 3-0 monofilament suture using the modified Allgöwer-Donati technique. The authors do not typically use a drain.

Postoperative Protocol

The postoperative protocol includes splint immobilization for 2 weeks, followed by serial cast immobilization for an additional 8 to 10 weeks. The patient is kept strictly non–weight-bearing for a total of 10 to 12 weeks postoperatively. The patient is then converted to a compression stocking and removable fracture boot, and progressive weight-bearing is commenced. The patient is gradually transitioned to regular

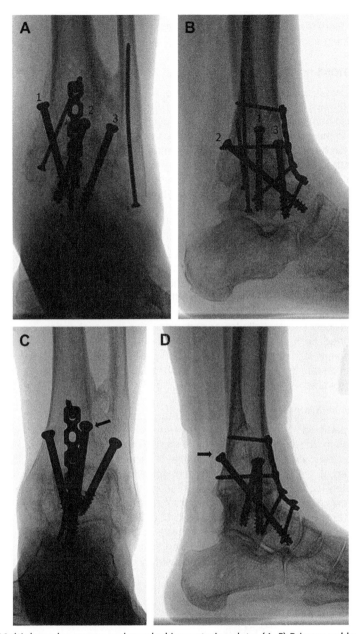

Fig. 4. Multiplanar lag screws and non-locking anterior plate. (*A–B*) Primary ankle arthrodesis for posttraumatic arthritis. (1) The medial screw is placed as vertically oriented as possible in both the coronal and sagittal planes to allow sufficient room for subsequent screws. (2) The posterior screw is placed parallel to the longitudinal axis of the talus in both the sagittal and transverse planes, stopping shy of the talonavicular joint. (3) The lateral screw is placed anterior to and divergent from the medial screw in sagittal plane. Note two screws from original fracture fixation. (*C–D*) Staged ankle arthrodesis for failed, infected total ankle arthroplasty. Note more vertical orientation of posterior screw to accommodate inlay graft (*black arrow*). Also note noncollinear tibial–hindfoot axis from subtle anterior translation.

shoe wear thereafter. Physical therapy is instituted on an individual basis as needed for gait training and strengthening exercises.

COMPLICATIONS
Malposition

In most instances, preservation of the fibula and the subchondral plate through use of the anatomic compression arthrodesis technique allows symmetric positioning of the ankle joint in the coronal plane such that varus or valgus malalignment is quite rare. Plantarflexion malalignment or uncorrected anterior translation of the talus, particularly in posttraumatic cases, is encountered more frequently. Precontoured locking plates may similarly have a tendency to anteriorly translate the talus in certain patients because of individual variations in anatomy. Both plantarflexion and anterior translation mechanically lengthen the foot, making it more difficult for the patient to vault over the top of the foot with gait (**Fig. 5**).

Arthrodesis Nonunion

Although nonunion rates are historically as high as 40%, most current ankle arthrodesis series using various rigid internal fixation techniques report nonunion rates of approximately 10% for low-risk patients with minimal deformity and adequate bone stock.[1] The increased stability provided by multiplanar lag screws and an anterior plate has yielded substantially lower nonunion rates in recent series. Kakarala and Rajan reported no nonunions among their subset of 11 ankle arthrodesis treated with multiplanar lag screws and an anterior plate.[13] Clare and colleagues[14] had a 4% nonunion rate in their large series, which included high-risk patients with significant comorbidities.

Implant Failure/Symptomatic Hardware

With this particular fixation strategy, the nonlocking anterior plate functions as a neutralization device, providing torsional protection to the multiplanar screws, and as a tension band device, countering cantilever bending forces in the sagittal plane. One or more of the anterior small fragment screws, particularly those in the talus, may ultimately loosen or fracture without affecting the overall stability of the multiplanar lag screws (**Fig. 6**). Clare and colleagues[14] reported loosening or failure of one or more of the anterior small fragment screws in 12 of 275 ankle arthrodeses (4.4%). They reported no correlation between screw fracture or lucency and union rate.

Positioning of the anterior plate too distal on the talus may lead to anterior impingement against the navicular body with compensatory dorsiflexion of the hindfoot during

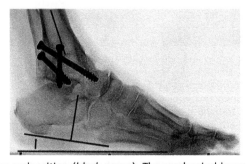

Fig. 5. Plantarflexion malposition (*black arrow*). The mechanical lever arm of the foot has been lengthened, impeding heel-to-toe vaulting with gait.

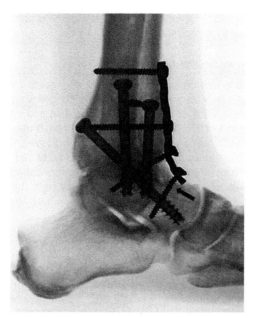

Fig. 6. Fracture of small fragment screw (*black arrow*) within anterior plate.

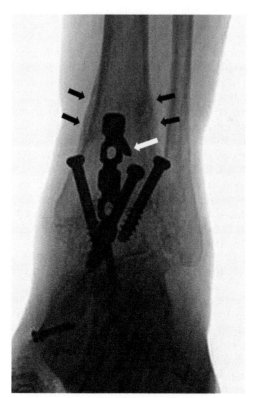

Fig. 7. Tibial stress fracture above the anterior plate (*black arrows*). Note the downward trajectory of the proximal-most screw within the plate (*white arrow*).

gait. Clare and colleagues[14] reported anterior impingement pain necessitating plate removal in 5 of 275 ankle arthrodeses (1.8%).

Tibial Stress Fractures above the Anterior Plate

Stress reaction or stress fractures in the distal tibia after ankle arthrodesis have been reported with multiple cancellous screws,[20] multiple cancellous screws and an anterior T plate,[21] and with a hindfoot arthrodesis nail.[22] Clare and colleagues[14] reported a tibial stress fracture in 4 of 275 (1.4%) ankle arthrodeses. These occurred with equal frequency with stainless steel and titanium implants; however, in all four cases, the proximal-most small fragment screw within the anterior plate had a slightly downward trajectory (**Fig. 7**). All four stress fractures resolved with protected weight-bearing in a fracture. They now diverge the proximal screw away from the plate proximally to lessen the stress riser effect of the anterior plate.

REFERENCES

1. Haddad SL, Coetzee JC, Estok R, et al. Intermediate and long-term outcomes of total ankle arthroplasty and ankle arthrodesis. J Bone Joint Surg Am 2007;89: 1899–905.
2. Davis RJ, Millis MB. Ankle arthrodesis in the management of traumatic ankle arthrosis: a long-term retrospective study. J Trauma 1980;20:674–8.
3. Helm R. The results of ankle arthrodesis. J Bone Joint Surg Br 1990;72:141–3.
4. Lynch AF, Bourne RB, Rorabeck CH. The long-term results of ankle arthrodesis. J Bone Joint Surg Br 1988;70:113–6.
5. Moeckel BH, Patterson BM, Inglis AE, et al. Ankle arthrodesis. A comparison of internal and external fixation. Clin Orthop 1991;268:78–83.
6. Holt ES, Hansen ST, Mayo KA, et al. Ankle arthrodesis using internal screw fixation. Clin Orthop 1991;268:21–8.
7. Maurer RC, Cimino WR, Cox CV, et al. Transarticular cross-screw fixation. A technique of ankle arthrodesis. Clin Orthop 1991;268:56–64.
8. Tarkin IS, Mormino MA, Clare MP, et al. Anterior plate supplementation increases ankle arthrodesis construct rigidity. Foot Ankle Int 2007;28:219–23.
9. Thordarson DB, Markolf K, Cracchiolo A III. Stability of an ankle arthrodesis fixed by cancellous-bone screws compared with that fixed by an external fixator. A biomechanical study. J Bone Joint Surg Am 1992;74:1050–5.
10. Thordarson DB, Markolf KL, Cracchiolo A III. Arthrodesis of the ankle with cancellous-bone screws and fibular strut graft. Biomechanical analysis. J Bone Joint Surg Am 1990;72:1359–63.
11. Chen YJ, Huang TJ, Shih HN, et al. Ankle arthrodesis with cross screw fixation. Good results in 36/40 cases followed 3–7 years. Acta Orthop Scand 1996;67: 473–8.
12. Mears DC, Gordon RG, Kann SE, et al. Ankle arthrodesis with an anterior tension plate. Clin Orthop 1991;268:70–7.
13. Kakarala G, Rajan DT. Comparative study of ankle arthrodesis using cross screw fixation versus anterior contoured plate plus cross screw fixation. Acta Orthop Belg 2006;72:716–21.
14. Clare MP, Swanson SA, Ketz JP, et al. Clinical results of the anatomic compression arthrodesis technique with anterior plate augmentation for ankle arthrodesis. Presented at American Orthopaedic Foot and Ankle Society, 25th Annual Summer Meeting. Vancouver, British Columbia (Canada), July 15–18, 2009.

15. Plaass C, Knupp M, Barg A, et al. Anterior double plating for rigid fixation of isolated tibiotalar arthrodesis. Foot Ankle Int 2009;30:631–9.
16. Guo C, Yan Z, Barfield WR, et al. Ankle arthrodesis using anatomically contoured anterior plate. Foot Ankle Int 2010;31:492–8.
17. Berkowitz MJ, Clare MP, Sanders RW, et al. The salvage of failed total ankle arthroplasty with conversion to ankle or ankle-hindfoot arthrodesis: results and techniques using structural allografts and internal fixation. Presented at American Orthopaedic Foot and Ankle Society, 25th Annual Summer Meeting. Vancouver, British Columbia (Canada), July 15–18, 2009.
18. Culpan P, Le Strat V, Piriou P, et al. Arthrodesis after failed total ankle replacement. J Bone Joint Surg Br 2007;89:1178–83.
19. Campbell CJ, Rinehart WT, Kalenak A. Arthrodesis of the ankle: deep inlay grafts with maximum cancellous-bone apposition. J Bone Joint Surg Am 1974;56: 63–70.
20. Lidor C, Ferris LR, Hall R, et al. Stress fracture of the tibia after arthrodesis of the ankle or the hindfoot. J Bone Joint Surg Am 1997;79:558–64.
21. Rowan R, Davey KJ. Ankle arthrodesis using an anterior AO T plate. J Bone Joint Surg Br 1999;81:113–6.
22. Thordarson DB, Chang D. Stress fractures and tibial cortical hypertrophy after tibiotalocalcaneal arthrodesis with an Intramedullary nail. Foot Ankle Int 1999; 20:497–500.

Open Posterior Approach for Tibiotalar Arthrodesis

Florian Nickisch, MD*, Frank R. Avilucea, MD, Timothy Beals, MD,
Charles Saltzman, MD

KEYWORDS

• Tibiotalar • Arthrodesis • Posterior approach

HISTORICAL PERSPECTIVE

Traumatic injury to the ankle and hindfoot often results in tibiotalar or subtalar arthritis. The associated joint pain, stiffness, and deformity may be difficult to treat with conservative measures. For such problems, arthrodesis of the ankle or hindfoot joints is the mainstay of treatment.

First described by Morgan and colleagues[1] in 1879, the operative principle of approximating and securing the talus and tibial plafond surfaces of viable cancellous bone to complete a tibiotalar arthrodesis has now been described by many researchers.[1–16] At present, surgeons use various techniques for the treatment of symptomatic tibiotalar arthrosis. In general, the technique used is determined by the underlying disorder, the presence and degree of deformity, the state of the soft tissue envelope, and patient factors, such as age, functional level, bone quality, previous surgeries, and medical comorbidities. Different techniques are used in patients with different characteristics; external fixators may be used for patients with septic arthritis or severe osteopenia, arthroscopic arthrodesis and percutaneous screw placement is used for those with minimal deformity, retrograde intramedullary nailing is done for those with concomitant subtalar arthritis, and open arthrodesis is often selected for patients with significant deformity. For open arthrodesis, various directional approaches have been described, including lateral transfibular approach with or without preservation of the distal fibula and anterior, anterolateral, and anteromedial (mini-open), and posterior approaches.[5,17–26] In the setting of a compromised soft tissue envelope, a posterior approach, through a single incision, often offers the healthiest and deepest soft tissue bed for reconstruction. This

The authors have nothing to disclose.
Department of Orthopaedics, University of Utah, 590 Wakara Way, Salt Lake City, UT 84108, USA
* Corresponding author.
E-mail address: Florian.Nickisch@hsc.utah.edu

approach is particularly useful in patients with previous medial, lateral, or anterior incisions from fracture fixation, ankle arthroplasty, or arthrodesis attempts.

In 1956, Staples[27] endorsed the posterior approach when the anterior soft tissue envelope is scarred, and there is concomitant need for talocalcaneal arthrodesis. Gruen and Mears[24] reported excellent and good results with the use of a blade plate to treat nonunion of the distal tibia, ankle, or subtalar joint through a posterior approach. Hanson and Cracchiolo[28] described the use of the posterior approach to place a 95° blade plate for a tibiotalocalcaneal (TTC) arthrodesis in patients with mild to moderate hindfoot deformity, failed fusion, and anterior soft tissue scarring secondary to previous surgery; each patient had a successful arthrodesis with this approach. To further assess potential complications, Hammit and colleagues[29] show that a midline posterior incision has a low primary wound complication rate. In addition, in their angiosome study assessing integument perfusion about the Achilles tendon, Yepes and colleagues[30] confirm that the posteromedial and posterolateral aspects of the ankle are well vascularized, with the watershed area localized to the posterior midline as previously described by Taylor and Pan.[31]

From a surgical technique standpoint, with the patient prone, the posterior approach grants the surgeon access to the entire posterior hindfoot and ankle. There is substantial exposure of each joint, so a large surface area may be surgically prepared for either a tibiotalar or TTC arthrodesis. Moreover, the unscarred tissue bed is deep and provides ample tissue for coverage of implants and bone graft. The prone position allows access to the posterior iliac crest for procurement of large bone grafts, if required. A posterior approach allows for the dissection necessary to mobilize large coronal plane deformities. Finally, by flexing the knee, hindfoot alignment is easily visualized in all planes and intraoperative images may be readily obtained because minimal foot manipulation is needed to obtain anteroposterior and lateral fluoroscopic images.

This article discusses the application of the posterior approach to complete, a tibiotalar and TTC arthrodeses as well as its use for converting a failed total ankle arthroplasty (TAA) to an arthrodesis.

INDICATIONS AND CONTRAINDICATIONS

The authors prefer the posterior approach as a salvage procedure when the anterior, medial, or lateral soft tissue envelope is compromised by previous injury, surgical intervention, or infection. Patients who are considered for this approach are typically those who have had a previous arthrodesis, have adjacent joint fusion or TAA and have progressed to either a symptomatic nonunion or implant failure requiring surgical revision (**Fig. 1**). This approach should be avoided in patients with poor vascular supply to the limb or if there is a need for anterior incisions or simultaneous foot surgery.

PRESURGICAL PLANNING

Revision surgery is indicated for patients with a painful nonunion or arthritis. It should be emphasized that treatment of nonunions is predicated on the reported symptoms. In evaluating the patient with previous ankle surgery, it is necessary to identify an accurate diagnosis, understand the cause of the pain, accurately identify the previous surgical interventions, and correlate that information with the mechanical findings of the physical examination and the appearance of radiographs before revision surgery is undertaken. Although a certain percentage of nonunions occur without a definite

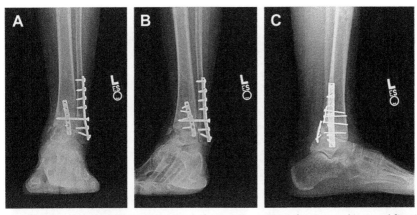

Fig. 1. A 50-year-old woman with a history of a revision open reduction and internal fixation of a pilon fracture after hardware failure. The 5-month postoperative radiographs demonstrate nonunion of posterior malleolus, hardware failure, and posttraumatic tibiotalar arthritis as seen on anteroposterior (*A*), mortise (*B*), and lateral (*C*) views.

cause, potential causes, such as infection or metabolic abnormalities, should be excluded and, if identified, treated before surgery.

A thorough history and physical examination begins the process of critically assessing the patient. Medical comorbidities, such as diabetes, peripheral neuropathy, rheumatoid arthritis, history of thromboembolic disease, or long-term use of steroids, must be discussed. Patients' skin is examined for previous traumatic and surgical scars and the quality of the soft tissue envelope is closely inspected. A complete neurovascular examination is essential to identify the quality of tissue perfusion as well as previous nerve injury. With nonpalpable pulses, the patient should be referred for a vascular consultation to establish whether arterial disease exists and, if so, whether a vascular intervention would improve tissue perfusion to promote healing and reduce the risk of infection. Previous nerve injuries must be discussed with the patient and documented so that there are no confusions about the cause of such deficits postoperatively. Sites of tenderness to palpation should be determined as well as the overall foot and ankle alignment, which should be compared with that of the contralateral limb. In cases of long-standing deformity, particular attention has to be paid to compensatory foot deformities. In a patient with a history of septic arthritis, wound healing problems, or previous postoperative infection, laboratory studies need to be reviewed to ensure resolution of any infectious process.

Each patient undergoes radiographic evaluation to include 3 weight-bearing views of both the ankle and foot along with a hindfoot alignment view.[32] In addition, a fine-cut (3 mm) computed tomographic (CT) scan of the ankle and hindfoot may be obtained to assess alignment, bone loss, and deformity, which may be difficult to discern on plain films. CT also allows the surgeon to inspect the integrity of adjacent joints and evaluate the available bone quality (**Fig. 2**) and is the gold standard for assessing the presence of union in patients with previous arthrodesis attempts.[33]

In discussing the risk of nonunion, it is important to ask about active tobacco use. Cigarette smoking is known to increase the risk for nonunion, and the patient should be encouraged strongly, if not convinced, to discontinue its use before and after surgical intervention, at least until the fusion is solidified.[34,35] Although no evidence clearly demonstrates improved union rates with perioperative smoking cessation, there is a trend for increased union rate when cigarette use is discontinued before

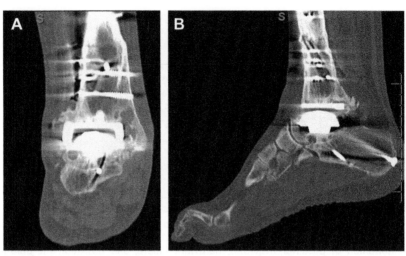

Fig. 2. Use of CT to examine bone stock quality. Coronal (*A*) and sagittal (*B*) views of a 63-year-old man's right ankle demonstrating failed tibiotalar arthroplasty with several lucencies surrounding tibial and talar components.

and after surgery.[35] In line with this notion, patients with rheumatoid disease should suspend immunosuppressant therapy 2 weeks preceding surgery.[36–38] Although there are limited data examining postoperative complications related to immunomodulatory therapy, methotrexate and tumor necrosis factor blockers are associated with an increased rate of infection.[36,38] Finally, diabetic patients are counseled regarding the importance of control of glucose levels throughout the perioperative period, and all patients, particularly those with several medical comorbidities, should have their nutrition optimized (albumin level <3.5 g/dL).

Many fixation options may be used for tibiotalar or extended hindfoot fusion through a posterior approach. In the authors' experience, the use of a posterior blade plate has resulted in relatively good success in many challenging situations, particularly for the indications that they describe. The authors place a 3.5-mm cannulated blade plate or fixed-angle device to provide rigid fixation of the arthrodesis. This implant is versatile in that it can be used for both tibiotalar and TTC arthrodeses. For tibiotalar fusion, a 90° blade plate is used, whereas for TTC arthrodesis the plate is usually opened to 100° to 110°. Because of the ease of contouring, the authors prefer a 3.5-mm to 4.5-mm plate. If a 4.5-mm plate is used, precontouring the plate before surgery reduces intraoperative tourniquet time. Supplementary large fragment screws are also used.

TECHNIQUE
Patient Positioning and Surgical Approach

After induction of general anesthetic, prophylactic antibiotics are administered. The authors prefer to place a pneumatic tourniquet about the thigh before positioning the patient prone on an image table with gel pads. The foot should rest off the table to allow ease of positioning. Two to three folded blankets are placed beneath the operative limb to elevate it above the contralateral leg so that anteroposterior and cross-lateral fluoroscopic images may be easily obtained. The entire operative limb and ipsilateral posterosuperior iliac spine are sterilized, prepared, and draped. Anatomic landmarks are palpated and marked directly over the Achilles tendon.

A 12- to 16-cm midline longitudinal incision exposes subcutaneous tissue, which is then sharply dissected down to the superficial fascia and paratenon overlying the Achilles tendon. These 2 layers are carefully cut longitudinally with the intent to preserve, reapproximate, and keep separated from superficial tissue at the time of closure. Careful dissection of the proximal wound is required to avoid injury to the small saphenous vein and sural nerve. To prevent compromising blood supply to the skin, the integrity between the paratenon, superficial fascia, and skin is maintained. Thus, during dissection, the surgeon should gently retract the skin, avoid excessive spreading with dissection scissors between these layers, and refrain from using self-retaining retractors.

A longitudinal tenotomy of the Achilles is completed taking care to create equal medial and lateral flaps. A tenotomy of the Achilles in the coronal plane, alternatively, may be completed so that the glistening layer of the tendon abuts paratenon when the wound is closed. Each flap is retracted with respective skin edges to enable visualization of the deep compartment (**Fig. 3**). On dissecting deep to the Achilles, the deep posterior compartment fascia is incised from distal to proximal longitudinally exposing the deep compartment musculature. The lateral aspect of the flexor hallucis longus (FHL) is identified, and the FHL and medial soft tissues are bluntly retracted medially after elevation of the lateral aspect of the FHL off the fibular periosteum and interosseous membrane; this step protects the neurovascular bundle in this muscular envelope and provides full exposure and access to the posterior tibia, ankle joint, subtalar joint, and distal fibula (**Fig. 4**). During this dissection, skin retractors are used only after deeper tissues are encountered. Moreover, care is taken to maintain full-thickness flaps to optimize vascular supply to the skin edges. Meticulous surgical technique throughout the procedure and prevention of excessive traction of skin preserves angiosomal circulation and helps prevent tissue breakdown, necrosis, and infection.

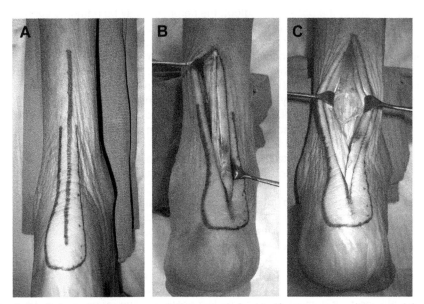

Fig. 3. (*A–C*) Posterior midline surgical approach for hindfoot exposure. (*Reprinted from* Ritter M, Nicksich F, DiGiovanni CW. Posterior bladeplate for salvage of failed total ankle arthroplasty. In: Wiese SW, editor. Operative techniques in orthopaedic surgery. Philadelphia: Wolters Kluwer/Lippincott Williams & Wilkins; 2010. p. 4211; with permission.)

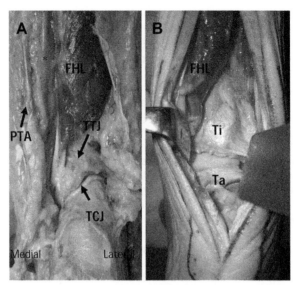

Fig. 4. (*A*, *B*) Deep compartment anatomy for hindfoot exposure. Asterisk indicates the tibial nerve. PTA, posterior tibial artery; Ta, talus; TCJ, talocalcaneal joint; Ti, tibia; TTJ, tibiotalar joint. (*Reprinted from* Ritter M, Nicksich F, DiGiovanni CW. Posterior bladeplate for salvage of failed total ankle arthroplasty. In: Wiese SW, editior. Operative techniques in orthopaedic surgery. Philadelphia: Wolters Kluwer/Lippincott Williams & Wilkins; 2010. p. 4208–9; with permission.)

Tibiotalar Arthrodesis

With full access to the posterior hindfoot, the peroneals may be retracted subperiosteally from the distal fibula to access the lateral gutter of the tibiotalar joint. Access to this part of the joint allows incorporation of larger joint surface area in the fusion mass in addition to a greater amount of bleeding bone to promote bone healing after physical approximation of the graft and native bone. The decision of whether to include the lateral gutter in the arthrodesis is based on the amount of degenerative disease, degree of deformity, length relationship of the tibia and fibula, and lastly surgeon preference. If the fibula is to be incorporated into the fusion, the authors typically perform a fibula osteotomy approximately 4 cm proximal to the tibiotalar joint line to uncouple the proximal fibula from the ankle; this osteotomy has been shown to improve distal tibiofibular fusion rates. Although this osteotomy may be performed through the posterior approach, it is often more easily accomplished through a separate lateral incision.

To prepare the tibiotalar joint for arthrodesis, a capsulotomy is initially performed. Part of the posterior malleolus is excised with an osteotome so that the posterior aspect of the tibia is flush with the posterior talus (**Fig. 5**), which not only improves visualization of the tibiotalar joint but also facilitates later placement of the blade plate; the excised piece of bone is morselized and saved for use as bone graft. In the setting of angular deformity, an osteotomy of distal tibia achieves angular correction (**Fig. 6**). Curettes, osteotomies, and rongeurs are used to remove articular cartilage from the distal tibia and talar dome. Lamina spreaders or Hintermann retractors may be used to distract the joint and improve access to the anterior aspect of the joint as well as the medial and lateral gutters. Once all cartilage is debrided and viable bone is visualized, the subchondral bone surfaces on the tibial and talar sides are perforated

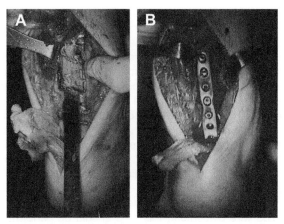

Fig. 5. Excision of posterior malleolus (*A*) to allow the plate to sit flush with the tibia and talus (*B*).

with several 2.5-mm drill holes to induce bleeding. The amount of bone required is determined, and structural or cancellous bone graft is harvested from the posterior iliac crest. The autograft is placed into the joint and firmly packed to evenly cover the entirety of the joint surface area. Structural graft may be necessary to fill large defects or correct deformities.

Blade plate application begins by positioning the foot in the desired alignment with 5° of valgus, neutral dorsiflexion, and slight external rotation. Reduction position is ascertained clinically and radiographically with fluoroscopy. The tibiotalar joint

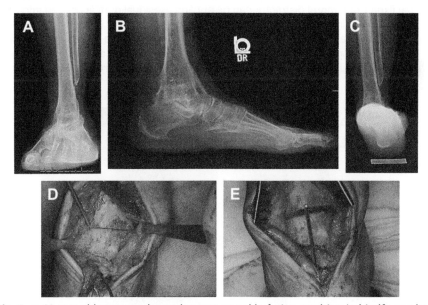

Fig. 6. A 60-year-old woman who underwent an ankle fusion resulting in hindfoot valgus and subtalar arthritis as seen on anteroposterior (*A*), lateral (*B*), and hindfoot alignment (*C*) plain radiographs. In performing a TTC arthrodesis through the posterior approach, the surgeon may also complete a supramalleolar osteotomy to correct such valgus deformity as shown in (*D*) and (*E*).

reduction can be secured with the placement of 2 Steinmann pins percutaneously from the medial tibial metaphysis. Alignment is verified clinically and with anteroposterior and lateral fluoroscopic images. The ideal entry point for the blade into the talar body is identified, typically a few millimeters proximal to the posterior facet of the subtalar joint. Correct positioning of the guide wire is critical. Because proximal exposure of the tibia is limited due to the bulk of the deep posterior compartment musculature, the hinged drill guide provided in the instrument set of the cannulated blade plate systems is impractical for this application. Instead the blade plate itself can be used as a guide by turning it 180°, so that the blade faces the surgeon. The plate is then placed flush on the posterior aspect of the distal tibia, and the guide wire is advanced into the talar body. The plate may need to be prebent to achieve greater or lesser dorsiflexion. Medial deviation of the talar neck must be accounted for when advancing the guide wire to prevent lateral penetration of the blade. The authors prefer using a custom-modified drill guide. Regardless of the method of guide wire placement, this step should be performed under fluoroscopic control in the lateral projection. Once the guide wire is in a satisfactory position in this plane, an anteroposterior fluoroscopic image of the foot is obtained to verify appropriate position in the talar neck (**Fig. 7**). The talus being dense, predrilling a trough into the it before plate insertion is strongly recommended to avoid fracture. The proper length and angle of the plate must be assessed to avoid cutout or penetration of the talonavicular joint and ensure appropriate positioning once the plate is set in its final position. Typically a 6- or 8-hole plate with a 35- to 45-mm blade is used. Serial images with fluoroscopy help the surgeon visualize the plate position. Before locking the plate in its final position with a single proximal and distal compressive screw, the foot and ankle position is evaluated clinically and radiographically to confirm proper alignment. If additional compression is desired, a large external fixator or femoral distractor can be applied. Residual graft is packed into and around the joint. Final radiographs are taken, and repeat clinical examination is done to ensure proper alignment. The deep-posterior musculature is laid over the plate, the Achilles is reapproximated and repaired, as is the paratenon and overlying superficial fascia, with closure of the remaining soft tissues in a layered manner.

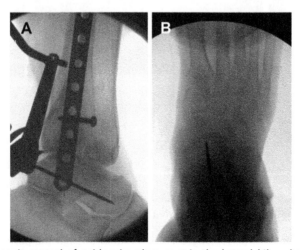

Fig. 7. Fluoroscopic control of guide wire placement in the lateral (*A*) and anteroposterior (*B*) projection is critical.

TTC Arthrodesis

Exposure of the tibia, talus, and os calcis follows the aforementioned surgical approach. After preparation of the tibiotalar joint, the subtalar joint is prepared similarly. As with the tibiotalar arthrodesis, the foot is aligned in 5° of valgus and external rotation. A Steinmann pin is inserted percutaneously from the plantar surface of the heel to the tibia to transfix the foot in the desired position; clinical examination and radiographs confirm position. The 3.5-mm or precontoured 4.5-mm 90° fixed-angle blade plate is laid in the anticipated position, and serial fluoroscopic images are taken so the plate may be adjusted to sit centrally along the TTC axis. Because of the soft cancellous bone of the calcaneus, it is not necessary to predrill a trough to introduce the plate into the calcaneus, but doing so may prevent inadvertent tracking of the plate. The starting position and angle for insertion of the blade into the calcaneus, however, requires careful attention because this starting point will determine apposition of bone to plate once the plate is seated in its final position. The blade should be close to the hard subchondral bone of the posterior facet to achieve greatest joint compression in the final construct. Once the plate is seated into the calcaneus and buttresses, the posterior hindfoot, plate position, and foot and ankle alignment is confirmed with anteroposterior and lateral radiographs before securing with screws. Additional bone graft is packed around the plate at the tibiotalar and subtalar joints. Reconstitution of the tendo Achilles and overlying soft tissue follows the procedure previously described for wound closure.

Failed TAA

TAA is commonly completed through an anterior approach. In settings in which TAA has failed and there is a need to convert to a tibiotalar arthrodesis, the posterior approach does not preclude the surgeon from removing this hardware. A femoral distractor or an external fixator with medial pins in the tibia and calcaneus facilitate joint distraction for straightforward implant removal. The remaining fibrous tissue and debris should be excised down to the bleeding trabecular bone. Alignment, bone graft requirement, and implant size needed for arthrodesis are determined. The tibiotalar or, occasionally, TTC arthrodesis procedure follows the same process as described previously.

COMPLICATIONS

There are limited reports in the literature discussing clinical outcome after fusion with a posterior blade plate.[24,28,29] In the authors' experience, patients have had generally satisfactory results, and this technique could be used for the above-mentioned indications because it is versatile, addresses a difficult problem, and is relatively facile to complete. As with any major fusion procedure, there are complications of this technique, such as stress fractures above the fixation and nonunion with hardware failure.

POSTOPERATIVE MANAGEMENT

Approximately 1 hour before surgical intervention, the patient administered a long-acting peripheral nerve block with an indwelling catheter placed under ultrasound guidance. In the authors' experience patients have experienced less postoperative nausea, constipation, and complications related to narcotic use and are more satisfied with pain control when regional anesthesia is administered.

Postoperatively, the patient's limb is initially placed in a very well-padded posterior U splint. If there is minimal bleeding, the splint is continued for 10 to 14 days and

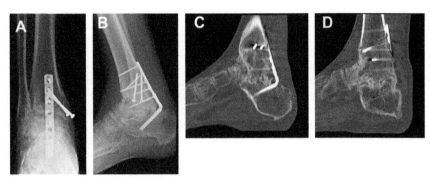

Fig. 8. A 27-year-old man who sustained a medial malleolus fracture and fracture-disloca-tion of his talus. After open reduction and internal fixation, the patient developed talar avascular necrosis and end-stage tibiotalar and subtalar arthritis. Patient underwent a TTC fusion. The 4-month anteroposterior (*A*) and lateral (*B*) radiographs demonstrate appro-priate hardware position, and the sagittal CT images (*C, D*) show near-complete tibiotalar joint fusion and subtalar fusion.

thereafter changed to a below-knee cast. In all other cases, the splint is changed to a below-knee cast on postoperative day 1 to 3. The limb is elevated for the first 2 to 5 days with pillows beneath the proximal calf, knee, and thigh, so that the distal leg is not in contact with any surface. Once in a cast, the patient remains non–weight-bearing for approximately 6 to 8 weeks. More precisely, weight bearing is restricted until there is radiographic evidence of trabecular bone bridging on plain radiographs or CT scan (**Fig. 8**). Thereafter, the patient's foot is placed in a boot, physical therapy is commenced, and weight bearing is slowly advanced, initially beginning with 25% of total weight with a weekly increase of 25% thereafter. On average, total length of partial weight bearing is 3 to 4 months. Lastly, rocker bottom shoes help the patient transition to shoe wear.

SUMMARY AND OUTLOOK

The posterior approach offers several advantages as a salvage technique. The use of a blade plate affords axial and rotational stability and the potential for compression. Compromised anterior soft tissue is avoided, and there is ample posterior soft tissue coverage of hardware and bone graft material. With the patient prone, all planes of ankle and foot alignment may be easily viewed clinically and with fluoroscopy, and access to the posterior iliac crest allows for a large volume of bone graft or bone marrow aspirate. In addition, access to the distal tibia, talus, and calcaneus is achieved with this incision, allowing for rigid fixation of the tibiotalar or TTC joints as well as enabling for removal of TAA implants.

REFERENCES

1. Morgan CD, Henke JA, Bailey RW, et al. Long-term results of tibiotalar arthrodesis. J Bone Joint Surg 1985;67:546–50.
2. Barr JS, Record EE. Arthrodesis of the ankle joint: indications, operative technic and clinical experience. N Engl J Med 1953;248:53–6.
3. Mann RA, Van Manen JW, Wapner K, et al. Ankle fusion. Clin Orthop 1991;268: 49–55.
4. Charnley J. Compression arthrodesis of the ankle and shoulder. J Bone Joint Surg Br 1951;33:180–91.

5. Ratliff AH. Compression arthrodesis of the ankle. J Bone Joint Surg Br 1959;41: 524–34.
6. Scranton PE Jr. Use of internal compression in arthrodesis of the ankle. J Bone Joint Surg Am 1985;67:550–5.
7. Wang GJ, Shen WJ, McLaughlin RE, et al. Transfibular compression arthrodesis of the ankle joint. Clin Orthop 1993;289:223–7.
8. Holt ES, Hansen ST, Mayo KA, et al. Ankle arthrodesis using internal screw fixation. Clin Orthop 1991;268:21–8.
9. Malarkey RF, Binski JC. Ankle arthrodesis with the Calandruccio frame and bimalleolar onlay grafting. Clin Orthop 1991;268:44–8.
10. Mears DC, Gordon RG, Kann SE, et al. Ankle arthrodesis with an anterior tension plate. Clin Orthop 1991;268:70–7.
11. Myerson MS, Quill G. Ankle arthrodesis. A comparison of an arthroscopic and an open method of treatment. Clin Orthop 1991;268:84–95.
12. Paremain GD, Miller SD, Myerson MS. Ankle arthrodesis: results after the miniarthrotomy technique. Foot Ankle Int 1996;17:247–52.
13. Thordarson DB, Markolf KL, Cracchiolo A III. External fixation in arthrodesis of the ankle: a biomechanical study comparing a unilateral frame with a modified transfixion frame. J Bone Joint Surg Am 1994;76:1541–4.
14. Newman A. Ankle fusion with the Hoffmann external fixation device. Foot Ankle 1980;1:102–9.
15. Kile TA, Donnelly RE, Gehrke JC, et al. Tibiocalcaneal arthrodesis with an intramedullary device. Foot Ankle Int 1994;15:669–73.
16. Moore TJ, Prince R, Pochatko D, et al. Retrograde intramedullary nailing for ankle arthrodesis. Foot Ankle Int 1995;16:433–6.
17. Mann RA. Arthrodesis of the foot and ankle. In: Coughlin MJ, Mann RA, Saltzman CL. Surgery of the foot and ankle. 8th edition. Philadelphia: Mosby Elsevier; 2007. p. 1087–125.
18. Horwitz T. The use of the transfibular approach in arthrodesis of the ankle joint. Am J Surg 1942;60:550–2.
19. Adams JC. Arthrodesis of the ankle joint: experiences with the transfibular approach. J Bone Joint Surg Br 1948;30:506–11.
20. Schuberth JM, Cheung C, Rush SM, et al. The medial malleolar approach for arthrodesis of the ankle: a report of 13 cases. J Foot Ankle Surg 2005;44:125–32.
21. Campbell CJ, Rinehart WT, Kalenak A. Arthrodesis of the ankle. J Bone Joint Surg 1974;56:63–70.
22. Chuinard EG, Peterson RE. Distraction–compression bone-graft arthrodesis of the ankle. J Bone Joint Surg 1963;45:481–90.
23. Hallock H. Arthrodesis of the ankle joint for old painful fractures. J Bone Joint Surg 1945;27:49–58.
24. Gruen GS, Mears DC. Arthrodesis of the ankle and subtalar joints. Clin Orthop 1991;268:15–20.
25. Morgan SJ, Thordarson DB, Shepherd LE. Salvage of tibial pilon fractures using fusion of the ankle with a 90 degree cannulated blade-plate: a preliminary report. Foot Ankle Int 1999;20:375–8.
26. Sward L, Hughes JS, Howell CJ, et al. Posterior internal compression arthrodesis of the ankle. J Bone Joint Surg Br 1992;74:752–6.
27. Staples OS. Posterior arthrodesis of the ankle and subtalar joints. J Bone Joint Surg 1956;38(1):50–83.
28. Hanson TW, Cracchiolo A. The use of a 95° blade plate and a posterior approach to achieve tibiotalocalcaneal arthrodesis. Foot Ankle Int 2002;23:704–10.

29. Hammit MD, Hobgood ER, Tarquinio TA. Midline posterior approach to the ankle and hindfoot. Foot Ankle Int 2006;27:711–5.
30. Yepes H, Tang M, Geddes C, et al. Digital vascular mapping of the integument about the Achilles tendon. J Bone Joint Surg 2010;92:1215–20.
31. Taylor GI, Pan WR. Angiosomes of the leg: anatomic study and clinical implications. Plast Reconstr Surg 1998;102:599–616.
32. Saltzman CL, El-Khoury GY. The hindfoot alignment view. Foot Ankle Int 1995;16:572–6.
33. Jones CP, Coughlin MJ, Shurnas PS. Prospective CT scan of hindfoot nonunions treated with revision surgery and low-intensity ultrasound stimulation. Foot Ankle Int 2006;27:229–35.
34. Cobb TK, Gabrielsen TA, Campbell DC, et al. Cigarette smoking and nonunion after ankle arthrodesis. Foot Ankle Int 1994;15(2):64–7.
35. Ishikawa SN, Murphy GA, Richardson EG. Effect of cigarette smoking on hindfoot fusions. Foot Ankle Int 2002;23(11):996–8.
36. Busti AJ, Hooper JS, Amaya CJ, et al. Effects of perioperative anti-inflammatory and immunomodulating therapy on surgical wound healing. Pharmacotherapy 2005;25(11):1566–91.
37. Pieringer H, Stuby U, Biesenbach G. Patients with rheumatoid arthritis undergoing surgery: how should we deal with antirheumatic treatment? Semin Arthritis Rheum 2007;36(5):278–86.
38. Ruyssen-Witrand A, Grossec L, Salliot C, et al. Complication rates of 127 surgical procedures performed in rheumatic patients receiving tumor necrosis factor alpha blockers. Clin Exp Rheumatol 2007;25:430–6.

Primary Tibiotalocalcaneal Arthrodesis

Kalpesh S. Shah, MS, FRCS (Tr&Orth)[a], Alastair S. Younger, ChM, MD[a,b],*

KEYWORDS

• Tibiotalocalcaneal • Arthrodesis • Retrograde • Nailing

Tibiotalocalcaneal (TTC) arthrodesis is a salvage procedure for severe arthritis and deformity of both the tibiotalar and subtalar joints (Canadian Orthopaedic Foot and Ankle Society [COFAS] grade 4).[1] For the purpose of this and other orthopedic articles, surgical arthrodesis of the ankle (tibiotalar) and subtalar (talocalcaneal) joints in the same operative sitting is termed TTC arthrodesis. Arthrodesis of the tibia to the calcaneus in the absence of the talus (such as extrusion/resorption) is termed as tibiocalcaneal (TC) arthrodesis. Arthrodesis of the talus to all the bones articulating with it (tibia, calcaneus, navicular, and cuboid) is termed pantalar arthrodesis and is outside the intended scope of this publication. A review of literature about TTC arthrodesis and the use of an intramedullary nail fixation to achieve TTC arthrodesis is presented. Intramedullary fixation is not the only method that can achieve TTC arthrodesis. Other alternatives are screws, plates, and external fixation. However, the use of an intramedullary device to achieve TTC arthrodesis has the advantages of providing immediate rigid internal fixation and compression at the arthrodesis site and offers load-sharing capacity. It is also useful in osteopenic bone, in which achieving solid screw fixation can be difficult.

HISTORICAL PERSPECTIVE

Arthrodesis of the tibia to the talus and the talus to the os calcis has been performed using posterior extra-articular methods described by Staples.[2] The earliest forms of modern day TTC arthrodesis were reported in 1906 when Lexer described a technique, which consisted of placing a boiled cadaver bone as a rod traversing through the tibia,

Grants: none.
The authors have nothing to disclose.
[a] Department of Foot and Ankle Surgery, St Paul's Hospital, 1081 Burrard Street, Vancouver, BC V6Z 1Y6, Canada
[b] Department of Foot and Ankle Surgery, University of British Columbia, Burrard Medical Centre, Suite 560-1144 Burrard Street, Vancouver, BC V6Z 2A5, Canada
* Corresponding author. Department of Foot and Ankle Surgery, St Paul's Hospital, 1081 Burrard Street, Vancouver, BC V6Z 1Y6, Canada.
E-mail address: asyounger@telus.net

Foot Ankle Clin N Am 16 (2011) 115–136
doi:10.1016/j.fcl.2010.12.001

talus and calcaneus.[3] Since then, numerous variations of this technique have been used. Ivory pegs, fibular grafts, metal spikes, and nails of various different forms have all been used in attempting TTC arthrodesis. In 1915 Albee[4] used the fibula as a vertical spike to perform an ankle and subtalar arthrodesis. Adams,[5] Leikkonen,[6] Kuntscher,[7] and Bingold[8] described techniques for TTC arthrodesis in the late 1940s and the mid 1950s. Decades later, the idea was revisited by Adams[5] in 1948 when a 3-flanged nail was driven from the calcaneus into the tibial shaft. Kuntscher[7] had the same idea in 1967 when he used a conical nail inserted in a retrograde manner from the calcaneus into the tibia for TTC arthrodesis. In 1994, Kile and colleagues[9] described using a straight, interlocked, intramedullary device that was a modification of the Johnson Nail (Smith & Nephew Richards Inc, Memphis, TN, USA). This nail was placed in a retrograde manner through a plantar incision. Since then, various nails not originally designed for TTC arthrodesis have been used. Examples include the proximal humeral nails used by Hammett and colleagues,[10] and femoral nails, which were used by Pinzur and Kelikian[11] Today, several medical device companies offer nails designed specifically for TTC arthrodesis, and there is no longer a need to modify intramedullary devices for use in TTC arthrodesis.

INDICATIONS AND CONTRAINDICATIONS
Indications

Generally, the indications for a TTC/TC arthrodesis with an intramedullary nail cover painful arthritic destruction of the ankle and subtalar joints irrespective of the cause. The nail can also be used in cases in which the cost of sacrificing the subtalar joint is offset by the benefit of the nail. In patients with an impaired bone quality (eg, in those with rheumatoid arthritis, diabetes, and neuroarthropathy),[12] the nail system has more rigid and stable fixation providing an advantage over crossed screws.

Further indications are the avascular necrosis of the talus, leading to a TC arthrodesis after talectomy or TTC arthrodesis after partial talar excision, salvage after failed or infected total ankle arthroplasty,[12] and pseudarthrosis after tibiotalar arthrodesis. In many cases, the bone loss of the distal tibia or dorsal talus is significant, requiring fixation beyond the talus and distal tibia that the nail offers. Arthritis of the ankle and subtalar joint in combination with a malunited or malaligned distal tibia fractures can also be addressed with a TTC arthrodesis and a tibia osteotomy. In these cases, all 3 levels (subtalar joint, ankle joint, and distal tibia) can be stabilized with a long locked intramedullary nail. Even Chopart amputations are suggested to be combined with a TTC arthrodesis to stabilize the hindfoot and prevent a pes equinus deformity.[13]

Absolute Contraindications

Absolute contraindications include an extremity with critical vascular disturbances or one that has a severe active infection.[9,14] Severe fixed deformities of the ankle, hindfoot, and distal tibia are relative contraindications for the closed nailing technique for TTC arthrodesis because of the difficulty encountered in obtaining a collinear reduction of the distal tibial tibia, talus, and calcaneus. However, if the advantages of such an implant prevail, an additional osteotomy of the distal tibia can be performed. An intact and asymptomatic mobile subtalar joint is a relative contraindication. If the subtalar joint is stiff, such as that occurring after previous trauma, the loss of subtalar motion will not be a major factor in the patient's outcome.

THE SURGICAL APPROACH TO RETROGRADE INTRAMEDULLARY NAILING

For TTC nailing, patients can be positioned supine, lateral, or prone, depending on surgeon preference and the approach required for deformity correction. A wide contoured thigh tourniquet (250 mm Hg) can be used.[15] The tourniquet should be deflated to ream the tibia or if the tourniquet time exceeds 120 minutes. In patients with partial avascular necrosis of the talus, it is also suggested to perform the operation without a tourniquet to allow the intraoperative assessment of cancellous bleeding. Disinfection and draping of the concerned leg must include the foot and the entire lower limb, including the knee joint. A single-shot antibiotic prophylaxis is provided routinely.

Several approaches have been described for TTC arthrodesis. These approaches can be considered as open, arthroscopic, or combined (open and arthroscopic). Open approaches can be lateral (transfibular lateral or anterolateral), posterior (posteromedial or posterolateral), or anterior. Any of these approaches can be combined with a separate medial incision to adequately prepare the medial side. The authors do not recommend the transfibular approach because this results in excessive dissection. Resection of the fibula results in dislocation of the peroneal tendons and sometimes allows excessive hindfoot eversion. The fibula also acts as a vascularized lateral strut for the fusion mass.

Instead, in the lateral approach, the fibula can be rotated out of the field by transecting the lateral collateral ligaments and mobilizing the syndesmosis and interosseous ligaments. If the fibula is too long for the fusion site, then the distal fibula can be resected parallel to the lateral side of the talus, allowing reapproximation and fixation. Some surgeons (Hanson and Cracchiolo,[16] Russotti and colleagues,[17] Thordarson and Chang[18]) have described the posterior approach (prone position) with reflection of the Achilles tendon. The skin incision can be medial (retracting the flexor hallucis laterally) or lateral (retracting the flexor hallucis muscle medially) to the Achilles tendon. The anterior approach uses the interval between the tibialis anterior and extensor hallucis longus tendons and gives a good access to the ankle joint. In this situation, the jigs for a total ankle arthroplasty can be used to create a parallel cut on the distal fibula. The medial and lateral malleolus can also be accessed from the anterior incision.

AUTHORS' PREFERRED APPROACH—OPEN PROCEDURE

The surgical approach is individualized for each patient based on previous incisions, existing deformity, and so forth; but for most patients, the authors prefer a combined approach, which is an open anterior approach to the ankle joint with a lateral arthrotomy for the subtalar joint. The fusion should be correctly aligned in all 3 planes of translation and rotation because malunion compromises outcomes.

The Anterior Approach

The patient is positioned supine on a standard operating table, with the hip on the surgical side elevated to allow access to the lateral ankle and subtalar joint. A longitudinal skin incision is made in the interval between the tibialis anterior and extensor hallucis longus tendons. After ankle joint synovectomy, the anterior border of the talus and the distal tibia is inspected, and osteophytes are resected (**Fig. 1**).

IN SITU ARTHRODESIS

If the arthrodesis can be performed in situ (minimal bone loss or deformity), the shape of both articulating surfaces is preserved, which can be achieved best with the help of chisels and curettes. Subchondral sclerosis is fissured with a chisel or awl. The use of a distractor (lamina spreader) is recommended to open up the ankle joint and access the medial and lateral aspects of the joint. This procedure is crucial to attain a proper alignment of the talus within the ankle mortise. Plantarflexion and dorsiflexion of the

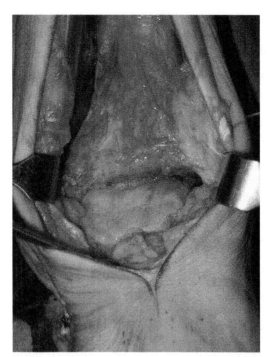

Fig. 1. Anterior arthrotomy of the ankle joint, showing good exposure of the joint.

ankle helps to expose the posterior and anterior portions of the talar dome. The exposure should allow removal of all cartilage in the joint, including that from the gutters and the posterior sides of the joint.

FLAT CUTS ON THE TIBIA AND TALUS

If there is bone loss, then the articular surface of the distal tibia and the superior articular surface of the talus is removed with a power saw perpendicular to the weight-bearing axis of the tibia. It is crucial to ensure that the cuts are correctly aligned. The tibial cut should be perpendicular to both axes of the tibia and the talar cut parallel to the floor with the foot in neutral standing position.

To achieve this result, the jigs for total ankle arthroplasty can be used with a minimal bone resection off the distal tibia. Alternatively, 2 Kirschner wires (K-wires) can be placed perpendicular to the axis in 2 planes. This positioning allows the surgeon to reference the cuts. The medial malleolus should be left intact to act as a buttress to control medial translation and internal rotation, which creates flush surfaces for compression and ideal positioning of the ankle for arthrodesis. The tips of both malleoli are trimmed back to facilitate compression. Bone graft is not used routinely but reserved for high-risk cases, such as avascular necrosis, nonunion defects, or diabetes.

In patients with avascular necrosis of the talus, a partial or total talectomy should be performed. To avoid marked length discrepancy, interposition of a well-molded corticocancellous bone graft (tissue bank) is recommended.

Preparation of the Subtalar Joint

The subtalar joint is approached from the lateral side under the tip of the fibula. Because the superior side of the talus has been dissected, care should be taken to avoid dissection into the sinus tarsi and into the vessels on the under surface of the talus.

A direct lateral approach under the tip of the fibula allows access of the joint and ensures complete debridement. The axis of the cone that forms the shape of the posterior facet can be seen and debrided of cartilage. In most cases, a subchondral dissection is performed. If there is bone loss, such as that after a calcaneal fracture, an interposition graft can be used.

ARTHROSCOPIC PROCEDURE

In some cases, the skin condition prevents an open approach. After trauma there may be compromise of the soft tissue envelope. In some patients with inflammatory arthropathies, prior wound healing issues indicate that an arthroscopic procedure is more advisable. In hemophilia (**Fig. 2**), an arthroscopic procedure may avoid bleeding complications. This procedure is not indicated in patients with severe bone loss or Charcot arthropathy.

Preparation of the Ankle Joint

The patient is positioned similar to the open procedure. A thigh tourniquet is used. The ankle joint is arthroscoped using a 2.9 high flow scope and cannula.

Most of the joint can be prepared using standard techniques. The anterior medial and anterior lateral portals allow most of the joint to be debrided. Curved curettes and osteotomes are invaluable to reach cartilage not accessible with a straight burr or abrader. An aggressive shaver is required. A burr with an auger to remove debris is very helpful and shortens the operating room time considerably. A posterior portal may often be necessary for the posterior debridement. The authors have used a direct medial approach with minimal complications but this has to be used with caution. Similarly a posterior lateral approach can be used but this is technically challenging from the supine position, and the surgeon should be aware of the position of the tibial

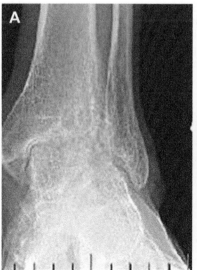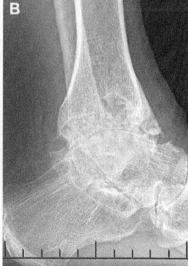

Fig. 2. (*A*) Hemophiliac arthropathy involving the ankle and subtalar joint: anteroposterior view. (*B*) Hemophiliac arthropathy involving the ankle and subtalar joint: lateral view.

nerve. All cartilage should be removed, including that from the gutters. The subchon-dral bone is prepared using a burr. After a complete debridement, the subtalar joint is prepared.

Preparation of the Subtalar Joint

For arthroscopy, a 2.9 scope may be tight for the subtalar fusion so a 1.9 or 2.4 scope should therefore be available. Otherwise the surgeon should have a 3.5 shaver and smaller curettes available. These devices usually fit both the ankle and subtalar joint. C-arm is essential for the procedure. After the ankle joint has been completely debrided, the subtalar joint is approached from the lateral portals. An anterior lateral, direct lateral, and posterior lateral portal is used. The foot is inverted to allow access while the surgeon sits on the lateral side of the table and works the portals of the sub-talar joint (**Fig. 3**). Sequential debridement of the posterior facet of the subtalar joint is performed using standard techniques (**Fig. 4**).

Nail Insertion

Once both joints have been debrided (open or arthroscopically), the instruments are withdrawn and the joints held in a neutral position. A retrograde nailing is the preferred method of fixation in these cases because its insertion can be minimally invasive and allows a strong mechanical construct. Reposition of the hindfoot is critically assessed (5° valgus, neutral dorsiplantar flexion, 5°–10° external rotation).

RETROGRADE NAILING—TECHNIQUE
Nail Designs

Some nails have a bend on the distal end, allowing a more lateral placement of the starting point in the calcaneus and potentially improving calcaneal fixation. Otherwise nail designs vary by the fixation achieved (lateral vs lateral and posterior screw fixation on the distal end), length (150–300 mm), and compression techniques. Compression may be achieved through the fusion site by dynamic proximal fixation. Distal fixation can be performed first, the nail impacted, and then proximal fixation performed. Alter-natively proximal fixation can be achieved first and then distal compression performed either on the nail or using an external compression device.

Regardless, the surgeon should perform some form of compression and should understand the nail system being used.

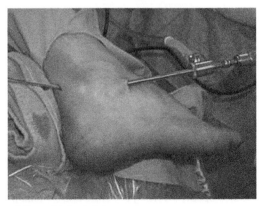

Fig. 3. Arthroscopy of the subtalar joint.

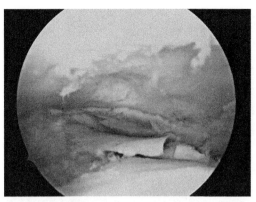

Fig. 4. Arthroscopic curettage of the subtalar joint: intraoperative view.

Screw configuration should also be considered when selecting a nail. Some nails are designed for normal talar bone stock. With bone loss, particularly in smaller patients, fixation can be hard to achieve or may make the nail prominent. More recent designs using fixation from the calcaneus obliquely into the talus address these issues. Proximal locking only controls rotation. The use of a locking screw in the tip of the nail, a requirement in fracture care, is not necessary unless a concomitant tibial osteotomy is performed.

Good product support is essential when using these nails because many surgeons in the operative team may be unfamiliar with its use. The product representative should be available for the case. It is worthwhile performing a cadaver or sawbones course before using a system such as this. The entry point in the calcaneus needs to be clearly understood because it is not intuitive. With a straight nail, the entry is on the medial slope of the anterior portion of the calcaneus.

Authors' preferred implant (**Fig. 5**)
    Material: Type 2 anodized titanium
    Side: left or right
    Aiming device: yes
    Compression: 5 mm
    Length: 150, 200, or 300 mm
    Diameter: 12 mm at base, 10/11/12 mm at the driving end (tip)
    Valgus: 5°
    Distal locking in calcaneus: lateral-medial and posteroanterior (this is rotated 10° from posteromedial to anterolateral plane)
    Distal locking talus: lateral-medial
    Proximal locking: 2 holes (1 dynamic, 1 static). The dynamic hole allows 5 mm axial movement.

Nail Entry Point

Traditionally, TTC nails have been a straight nail design. With straight nail designs, it can be difficult to achieve 5° of valgus. Attempts to achieve valgus with a straight nail can lead to an overly medial starting hole that can result in medial cut-out of the nail through the calcaneus. Conversely, a starting point with good bony support may be too lateral and may place the ankle in varus or position the nail at a high nail-tibial angle, leading to stress reaction or fracture.

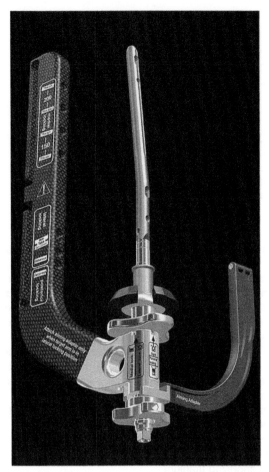

Fig. 5. Example of 1 of the nails designed for TTC arthrodesis. (*Courtesy of* Stryker, Inc. Mahwah, NJ; with permission.)

An incision is made on the plantar aspect of the foot directly in line with the long axis of the tibia with the foot in the corrected position. The starting point can be confirmed on anteroposterior and lateral image views before the incision being made and should be vertically underneath the long axis of the tibia with the ankle in a neutral position. The starting point is usually 1 to 2 cm behind the calcaneocuboid joint and on the medial slope of the calcaneus (**Fig. 6**). Care should be taken when exposing this part of the calcaneus from the plantar side to ensure that the tibial nerve is not damaged. The nerve lies on the medial side of the approach. Deep dissection should be performed bluntly and the medial soft tissues retracted.

Instrumentation

Once dissection is carried down to the calcaneus, the soft tissues are protected with Hohmann retractors; a K-wire is then inserted up through the calcaneus and into the central aspect of the tibia. An off-centered wire results in malreduction of the joint during insertion of the nail. For example, if the wire hits the anterior cortex and bends,

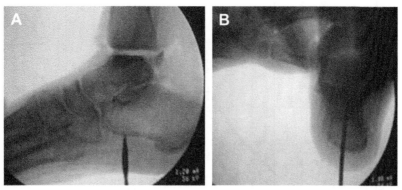

Fig. 6. (*A*) Nail entry point: anteroposterior view (intraoperative). (*B*) Nail entry point: axial view (intraoperative).

then reaming the calcaneus and talus in this position results in a greater degree of flexion than anticipated. Similarly, extension occurs if the wire hits the posterior cortex.

The position of the K-wire should be confirmed on the anteroposterior and lateral ankle views fluoroscopically. A stepped drill is passed over the K-wire and drilled up to the articulating surface of distal tibia, followed by passing of a ball-tipped guide wire through the reamed canal into the shaft of the tibia. The position of the guide

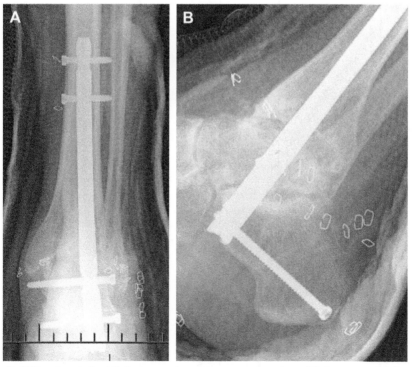

Fig. 7. TTC arthrodesis. (*A*) Postoperative anteroposterior view. (*B*) Postoperative lateral view.

Table 1
Clinical studies on TTC arthrodesis

Author	No. of Procedures	Mean Age (in y)	Indications for Surgery	Mean Follow-up (in mo)	Technique Used	Bone Graft Used	Implant Used	% Union	Mean Time to Union	% Satisfied	Conclusion
Gavaskar and Chowdary,[35] JOS 2009	7	40	TB Ankle	24	Arthroscopy assisted	No	Retrograde supracondylar femoral nail (Sharma Surgical & Engg. Pvt Ltd, Vadodara, Gujarat, India)	100	13 wk	Not given	TTC arthrodesis using a supracondylar femoral nail, combined with debridement and multidrug therapy, enabled a reliable 1-stage solution for advanced osteoarticular tuberculosis and early return to function.
Nagappa and Wood,[36] Foot 2007	11	55	RA	20	Anterior approach, preserve both malleoli for rotational stability	No	VersaNail (DePuy Inc, Warsaw, IN, USA)	82	Not given	Not given	TTC arthrodesis using a VersaNail and anterior approach is an effective procedure in RA.
Niinimaki et al,[37] FAI 2007	34	57	RA: 10 PTA: 10 ECV: 6 OA: 4 Charcot: 1 Other: 3	24	Transfibular	Fibula	Biomet Ankle fusion nail (Biomet Finland Oy, Koivuhaantie, Vantaa, Finland) with 1 PA screw	76	16 wk	90	TTC arthrodesis with a compressive retrograde intramedullary nail is safe and effective as a salvage procedure for patients with severe malalignment or arthrosis of the hindfoot
Ahmad et al,[38] FAI 2007	18	54.2	Charcot: 6 Neuromuscular: 3 PTA: 4 AVNT: 2 Inflam: 2	21.9	Transfibular	No	PHILOS plate (AO)	94.4	20.7 wk	82.4	PHILOS plate can offer an advantage (highly rigid fixation, easier to use) over blade plates in achieving TTC arthrodesis in patients with poor bone quality
Boer et al,[39] CORR 2007	50	57.6	PTA: 23 OA: 9 FTAR: 3 ECV: 9 FPS: 3	51	Transfibular, with percutaneous or open ankle debride, but no debride of STJ	Fibula	Orthofix nail with PA screws	96	20 wk	92	TTC arthrodesis with a retrograde intramedullary nail without formal debridement of the subtalar joint and with percutaneous debridement of the ankle in slightly greater than half of the cases is a reliable way of

Pelton et al,[40] FAI 2006	33	54	Charcot: 10 AVNT: 5 OA: 4 PTA: 8 Inflam: 2 CMT: 1 ECV: 2	14	Transfibular, with medial incision for medial malleolar resection	Fibula in most, iliac crest or femoral head in some	ACE VersaNail; straight with 2 PA locking	88	16 wk	82	TTC arthrodesis with dynamic retrograde intramedullary nailing is a good method of stabilizing this complex fusion construct.
Goebel et al,[41] JFAS 2006	29	54	OA RA PTA	40	Transfibular	No	Retrograde femur nail (Stryker, Kalamazoo, MI, USA)	90	25 mo	79	TTC arthrodesis using a retrograde intramedullay nail is an effective technique in achieving a solid fusion, relief from paini and improvement of quality of life
Komarasamy et al,[42] JBJSB Sup 2005	42	63	OA PTA RA	10	Transfibular	Fibula	Retrograde nail	67	Not given	62.5	TTC arthrodesis using an intramedullary nail remains a viable option in the management of concurrent ankle and subtalar joint arthritis, but patients should be warned of the potential for nonunion and high complication rates.
Hammett et al,[43] FAI 2005	52	57.1	Inflam: 11 OA: 5 PTA: 9 ECV: 6 Ankle mal/nu: 5 FTAR: 4 Charcot: 2 CMT: 4 Other neuropathies (polio, CP, foot drop): 6	34	Anterolateral in majority	Local, fibula, iliac crest, or femoral head	ACE Humeral (Biomet) nail	87	17 wk	82	TTC arthrodesis with intramedullary nailing is an effective technique for treating complex foot deformities and often is the only alternative to amputation.

(continued on next page)

Table 1
(continued)

Author	No. of Procedures	Mean Age (in y)	Indications for Surgery	Mean Follow-up (in mo)	Technique Used	Bone Graft Used	Implant Used	% Union	Mean Time to Union	% Satisfied	Conclusion
Anderson et al,[44] Acta Orthop 2005	25	56.6	RA	40.9	Transfibular	Fibula	5 designs of nail	96	Not given	92	TTC arthrodesis with retrograde intramedullary nail in patients with RA results in high rate of healing, a high rate of patient satisfaction, and relatively few complications.
Mendicino et al,[45] JFAS 2004	20	56	DMN: 7, OA: 4, PTA: 2, ECV: 2, RA: 2, Gout: 2, Ankle malunion: 1	19.8	Transfibular + medial malleolar resection	Fibula	First/Second generation (Smith & Nephew Richards Inc/ Biomet/DePuy)	95	4.1 mo	Not given	TTC arthrodesis with retrograde intramedullary nailing is a useful procedure for limb salvage in both diabetic and nondiabetic patients with gross instability or fixed deformity.
Millett et al,[46] Am J Ortho 2002	15	52	OA, PTA	24	Transfibular	Fibula	Retro nail	93.5	16.5 wk	93	TTC arthrodesis using a retrograde nail is an effective salvage technique in complex posttraumatic or postsurgical settings.
Hanson and Cracchiolo,[16] FAI 2002	10	64	PTA: 6, OA: 2, RA: 1, Postpolio deformity: 1	37	Prone position, posterior approach	Posterior iliac crest	95° angled blade plate (Synthes, West Chester, PA, USA)	100	14.7 wk	Good	TTC arthrodesis using a posterior approach, blade plate and bone grafts resulted in a solid fusion in all patients. This method is particularly effective in large patients with a mild-moderate hindfoot deformity.

Study											
Ebraheim et al,[47] CORR 2001	4	PTA with osteopenia	49.7	28	Fibula used as intramedullary graft	Fibula	K-wires, cannulated screws.	100	4 mo	100	TTC arthrodesis using an intramedullary fibular graft is less invasive than a intramedullary nail, provides both osteogenesis and fixation, and is useful for revision of failed arthrodesis in which an intramedullary nail was used for fixation.
Acosta et al,[48] FAI 2000	13	RA: 5 PTA: 4 OA: 2 CMT: 2	60	55 (14–59)	Transfibular but fibula split longitudinally and never excised so foot becomes narrow. The medial side of split fibula used as an onlay graft (calcaneus-tibia) or posterior with release of Achilles tendon	Fibular, iliac crest, or allograft	Ex Fx: 2 Cancellous bone screws: 8, 95° blade plate: 3 (posterior approach)	100	Not given	Not given	TTC arthrodesis is a useful salvage operation for treating advanced arthritic deformities of the ankle and hindfoot.
Chou et al,[49] FAI 2000	56	PTA:14 FPS: 12 OA: 11 AVNT: 7 RA: 6 FTAR: 2 Charcot: 2 CMT: 2	53	26	Transfibular	Fibula/Iliac crest/Allograft	Retro Nail: 37 Screws: 17 Plate: 1	86	19 wk	87	TTC arthrodesis is an effective salvage procedure for patients with disease both involving the ankle and subtalar joint.
Thordarson and Chang,[18] FAI 1999	12	Failed ankle fusion: 6 AVNT: 2 RA: 1 OA: 1 Charcot: 1 FTAR: 1	50	19.6	Lateral or posterior	Fibula/Iliac crest	ACE AIM nail.	100	Not given	Not given	TTC arthrodesis using intramedullary nail results in a stress reaction between the proximal locking screws in a significant number of patients.

(continued on next page)

Table 1 (continued)										
Author	No. of Procedures	Mean Age (in y)	Indications for Surgery	Mean Follow-up (in mo)	Technique Used	Bone Graft Used	Implant Used	% Union	Mean Time to Union	% Satisfied	Conclusion
Kile et al,[9] FAI 1994	30	48	OA PTA RA	4–27	Posterior	Iliac crest	Intramedullary nail.	90	Not given	87	TTC arthrodesis using an intramedullary nail gave satisfactory results in 87% of cases.
Papa and Myerson,[50] JBJSA 1992	13	45	PTA: 13	32	Transfibular. Second incision over MM to excise it	Fibula	Synthes can cancellous bone screws.	86	14 wk	Not given	TTC arthrodesis is a complex, technically demanding procedure, and should be regarded as a salvage operation capable of producing a satisfactory result and usually providing a reasonable alternative to amputation.
Russotti et al,[17] JBJS 1988	21	50	FPS: 8 FTAR: 5 AVNT: 4 No. of malunions: 2 Neuropathy: 2	49	Posterolateral	Iliac crest	External Fixator + Steinman pin.	86	Not given	75	TTC arthrodesis using a Steinmann pin or external fixator gave satisfactory results in 75% of cases.

Abbreviations: AAN, ankle arthrodesis nail; BMD, bone mineral density; Ex Fix, external fixator; FFC, fresh frozen cadaver; FPS, failed previous surgery; HAN, hindfoot arthrodesis nail; IMN, intramedullary nail; Inflam, inflammatory; mm, millimeter; Pt, patient; LM, lateral to medial; RA, rheumatoid arthritis; vs, versus.

wire in the center of the tibial canal should be confirmed with anteroposterior and lateral fluoroscopic views. The stepped drill is again passed over the guide wire and is used to open the tibial canal by drilling into the metaphyseal region of the tibia. The tibia should be sequentially reamed until appropriate cortical chatter is obtained. The nail is sized for 1 mm less than the last reamer diameter. The reamer should be passed beyond the planned length of the nail to ensure that the nail does not bind in the tibia before being fully seated. The tourniquet should be deflated for this part of the procedure to prevent heat necrosis of bone with dull reamers.

Nail Insertion

Before the insertion of the implant, the position of the foot is assessed again. Using the trial sizer, the length of the nail and the position of the distal locking screws can be monitored fluoroscopically. The intramedullary guide wire is removed. The appropriate nail is then firmly attached to the targeting device. Before the insertion, it should be confirmed that the nail holes match with the carriages for distal and proximal locking. With the jig usually running on the lateral side, the nail is inserted manually by mallet taps on the hammer pad. Depending on the foot deformity, it is also possible to advance the distal locking screws from the medial side. Again, intermittent fluoroscopic imaging is compulsory to ensure a correct implant position. The nail should advance continuously without any signs of mechanical conflict. If the surgeon feels any resistance during impaction, it is strictly suggested to remove the nail and repeat the reaming process. After fully advancing the nail, the end of the implant should be flushed with the plantar calcaneal surface to avoid any impingement. However, the end of the implant can either be left somewhat prominent (<5 mm) or advanced below the plantar cortex to allow ideal positioning of the locking screws.

Distal Locking

Distal locking can be attained with 2 or 3 screws. Ideal stability is achieved with both distal screws inserted in the os calcis and the third screw running into the talar body. Because most indications for intramedullary fixation of a TTC arthrodesis refers to severe hindfoot deformities, the loss of bone structure does often prevent the insertion of more than 1 calcaneal screw. At least 1 of the distal holes match with the os calcis, the proximal one with the talus. In patients with a TC arthrodesis, both distal screws can be advanced to the os calcis, whereas the third nail hole matches with the distal tibia. Depending on the anatomic situation and the bone quality, the locking screws are usually inserted from lateral to medial or from posterior to anterior. If the surgeon has decided to interpose a solid bone graft, this should be done before advancing the locking screw into the talus or the distal tibia.

Proximal Locking

Proximal locking can be dynamic or static fixation in the lateromedial or posteroanterior direction.

End Cap

Before the removal of the targeting device, fluoroscopic control should be performed in 2 planes to ensure proper implant position and appropriate screw length. Some nails offer an end cap for insertion into the distal tip of the nail.

The wounds are closed in layers and the patient immobilized in a plaster splint during the postoperative period. C-arm views are obtained at the end of the procedure (**Fig. 7**).

Table 2
Biomechanical studies about TTC arthrodesis

Author	No	Age	Experimental Condition	Objectives	Implant	Conclusion
Yakacki et al,[19] 2010	Synthetic bone and 2 cadavers	63, 66	2 types of retro IMN vs 2 types of circular frame.	Quantify compression forces of IMN and Ex Fx with respect to loading and simulated bone resorption (over the course of healing in a clinical situation).	Not given	Ex Fx capable of applying and sustaining greater amounts of compression due to application of force from wire bending. IMNs are capable of generating compression; however, they exhibit 90% decrease in compressive load with less than 1 mm of resorption.
Klos et al,[20] 2009	7 pairs FFC	77 (68–85)	Synthes HAN with 1 conventional screw and 1 locked spiral blade in calcaneus vs 1 conventional screw and 1 locked screw.	Compare rigidity in bending and torsion between the 2 constructs.	Not given	Screw + spiral blade stiffer in dorsiflexion/plantarflexion in early cyclic phase. No other difference between the 2. Screw + spiral blade should be considered when only the most distal IMN locking site can be used or in Pt requiring greater stability.
Santangelo et al,[21] 2008	10 pairs FFC	59 (32–86)	Retro IMN with 2 LM screws (1 calcaneus, 1 talus) vs circular ring fixator.	Compare bending and torsional stiffness of the 2 constructs.	Not given	Circular frame stiffer in torsion, but no difference in bending stiffness between the 2.
Muckley et al,[22] 2008	Synthetic bone and FFC (total 24 including 8 pairs)	Not given	Stryker T2 AAN (angle-stable locking nail) locked in dynamic compression proximally with and without compression (both internal and external) with Biomet arthrodesis nail in static locking (straight nail, no compression applied).	Compare initial stability and stability after cyclical loading.	Retro IMN	Angle-stable locking nails (with and without compression) had better initial stability as well as after cyclical loading. No significant difference observed with compression.

Study	Model	Age	Construct	Purpose		Results
Chodos et al,[23] 2008	9 pairs FFC	81 (63–99)	Locking plate vs blade plate.	Compare bending and torsional stiffness (initial and final), load-to-failure, fatigue endurance, and construct deformation.	Not given	Locking plates had higher initial stiffness, higher dorsiflexion and torsional load-to-failure, and lower construct deformation. Fixation with locking plate superior to that of blade plate.
O'Neill et al,[24] 2008	6 pairs FFC	78 (64–91)	10-hole lateral locking plate with TTC fusion screw (long p part threaded cannulated cancellous-calcaneus to tibia) vs Retro IMN with PA screw.	Compare dorsiflexion stiffness (initial and final), deformation and load-to-failure between the 2 constructs.	Not given	Locking plate superior to IMN in 3 of 4 parameters (except final stiffness).
Muckley et al,[25] 2007	Composite bone models; 3 for each device	Not given	Biomet nail (static locking mode and compressed mode), a Stryker T2 femoral nail (compressed mode); a prototype IM nail 1 (PT1, compressed mode), a prototype IM nail 2 (PT2, dynamic locking mode and compressed mode), and a 3-screw construct.	Compare contact surface area and primary stability of TTC arthrodesis construct using compressed and uncompressed retro IMNs with screws.	Not given	IMNs with compression were superior to uncompressed nails and screw construct with respect to contact area and primary stiffness.
O'Neill et al,[26] 2007	6 pairs FFC	Not given	Retro IMN with PA screw vs same with additional TTC fusion screw (long part threaded cannulated cancellous from calcaneous to tibia).	Compare dorsiflexion (initial and final) stiffness, load-to-failure, and construct deformation.	Not given	Initial and final stiffness and load-to-failure is higher with IMN + TTC arthrodesis augmented screw. Added screw provides more stable fixation.

(continued on next page)

Table 2
(continued)

Author	No	Age	Experimental Condition	Objectives	Implant	Conclusion
Means et al,[27] 2006	8 pairs FFC	70.5 (62–77)	LM (lateral to medial) screw vs PA screw with retrograde IMN.	Compare dorsiflexion stiffness (initial and final), load-to-fatigue, fatigue endurance, and plastic deformation between the 2 constructs.	Retro IMN	Retro IMN with PA screw provided more stable fixation than LM screw.
Noonan et al,[28] 2005	5 pairs FFC	70.4 ± 6.9	Retro IM Ankle fusion nails (standard length) vs Custom-made long retro IMN (ending at upper tibial metaphyses).	Measure mechanical strain along the tibia after TTC arthrodesis using the 2 devices.	Not given	Successful TTC arthrodesis with standard-length IMN creates a stress concentration around proximal screw holes, and this can be alleviated in Pt with generalized or localized osteopenia by using longer IMN that end in proximal tibial metaphyses.
Bennett et al,[29] 2005	Synthetic bone	Not given	3 crossed cancellous screws, 2 crossed cancellous screws, retro IMN (2 screws in calcaneous, 1 in talus), retro IMN with above-mentioned configuration with single tibiotalar bone staple.	Compare micromotion at the fusion site between different constructs.	Not given	3 crossed screw technique provided the greatest stability. Augmentation of retro IMN with single staple confers stability nearly equal to that of 3 crossed screws.
Alfahd et al,[30] 2005	7 pairs FFC	80 ± 8	Retro IMN vs Blade plate.	Compare bending and torsional (initial) rigidity and effect of BMD on stability using the 2 devices.	Not given	No difference between the 2 devices for the 2 parameters. Implant choice is a matter of surgeon preference or soft tissue status.

Study	Specimens		Construct	Purpose	BMD	Findings
Chiodo et al,[31] 2003	10 pairs FFC	Not given	DePuy AIM nail with 2 distal screws (1 in calcaneus, 1 in talus) vs Blade plate + single long part threaded cancellous screw (calcaneus to tibia).	Compare bending stiffness (initial and final), plastic deformation, and fatigue endurance between the 2 devices.	Not given	Higher initial and final stiffness and decreased plastic deformation in blade plate compared with nail. As BMD decreased, greater deformation was observed in nail group compared with blade plate group. This finding supports the use of blade plate in osteopenic bone.
Berson et al,[32] 2002	4 pairs FFC	Not given	First-generation nail with manual compression, Ex fix for compression with first-generation nail, Ex fix for compression with second-generation nail, nail-mounted compression device with second-generation nail.	Find the most reliable method to apply and maintain compression across the ankle joint.	Not given	Both Ex Fix and nail-mounted compression device produced compression, but significant compression was maintained only with the nail-mounted compression device.
Mann et al,[33,34] 2001	5 pairs FFC	Not given	Biomet AAN with transverse calcaneal screw (first-generation nail) and Biomet AAN nail with PA calcaneal screw (second-generation nail).	Compare rotational stability between the 2 constructs.	Not given	PA screw construct significantly stiffer in rotation.

Abbreviations: AAN, ankle arthrodesis nail; BMD, bone mineral density; Ex Fix, external fixator; FFC, fresh frozen cadaver; HAN, hindfoot arthrodesis nail; IMN, intramedullary nail; LM, lateral to medial; PA, posteroanterior; Pt, patient; vs, versus.

POSTOPERATIVE MANAGEMENT

Patients are observed at follow-up 7 to 10 days after surgery for removal of the splint and sutures. They are then placed into a circumferential fiberglass cast. Patients are instructed to be strictly non–weight bearing on the operative extremity until radiographic union is achieved. This period is ideally 4 to 6 weeks; however, in diabetic and neuropathic patients, in whom this procedure is often performed, the non–weight-bearing period can be 12 weeks or more. Once union is achieved, gradual weight bearing in a walking boot is allowed, and the patient is eventually transitioned out of the boot after 1 month. Long-term bracing is recommended for neuropathic patients undergoing this procedure even if solid arthrodesis is obtained to offload stress to the unfused midfoot and hindfoot joints.

Outcomes

See **Tables 1** and **2**.

REFERENCES

1. Krause FG, Di Silvestro M, Penner MJ, et al. Inter- and intraobserver reliability of the COFAS end-stage ankle arthritis classification system. Foot Ankle Int 2010; 31(2):103–8.
2. Staples OS. Posterior arthrodesis of the ankle and subtalar joints. J Bone Joint Surg Am 1956;38(1):50–8.
3. Boyd HB, Knight RA. Fractures of the astragalus. South Med J 1942;35:160–7.
4. Albee FH. Bone graft surgery. Philadelphia and London: W.B. Saunders; 1915. p. 335.
5. Adams JC. Arthrodesis of the ankle joint. Experiences with the transfibular approach. J Bone Joint Surg Br 1948;30:506–11.
6. Bingold AC. Ankle and subtalar fusion by a transarticular graft. J Bone Joint Surg Br 1956;38:862–70.
7. Kuntscher G. Combined arthrodesis of the ankle and sub-talar joints. In: Practice of intramedullary nailing. Springfield (IL): Charles C. Thomas; 1967. p. 207–9.
8. Leikkonen O. Astragalectomy as an ankle-stabilizing operation in infantile paralysis sequelae. Acta Chir Scand Suppl 1948;152:13–4.
9. Kile TA, Donnelly RE, Gehrke JC, et al. Tibiotalocalcaneal arthrodesis with an intramedullary device. Foot Ankle Int 1994;15:669–73.
10. Hammet R, Hepple S, Forster B, et al. Tibiotalocancaneal (hindfoot) arthrodesis by retrograde intramedullary nailing using a curved locking nail. The results of 52 procedures. Foot Ankle Int 2005;26:810–5.
11. Pinzur MS, Kelikian A. Charcot ankle fusion with a retrograde locked intramedullary nail. Foot Ankle Int 1997;18:699–703.
12. Hopgood P, Kumar R, Wood PL. Ankle arthrodesis for failed total ankle replacement. J Bone Joint Surg Br 2006;88:1032–8.
13. De Gere MW, Grady JF. A modification with Chopart's amputation with ankle and subtalar arthrodesis by using an intramedullary nail. J Foot Ankle Surg 2005;44: 281–6.
14. Cierny G, Cook G, Mader J. Ankle arthrodesis in the presence of ongoing sepsis. Orthop Clin North Am 1989;20:709–21.
15. Younger AS, McEwen JA, Inkpen K. Wide contoured thigh cuffs and automated limb occlusion measurements allow lower tourniquet pressures. Clin Orthop Relat Res 2004;428:286–93.

16. Hanson TW, Cracchiolo A. The use of a 95 degree blade plate and a posterior approach to achieve tibiotalocalcaneal arthrodesis. Foot Ankle Int 2002;23(8): 704–10.

17. Russotti GM, Johnson KA, Cass JR. Tibiotalocalcaneal arthrodesis for arthritis and deformity of the hind part of the foot. J Bone Joint Surg Am 1988;70(9): 1304–7.

18. Thordarson DB, Chang D. Stress fractures and tibial cortical hypertrophy after tibiotalocalcaneal arthrodesis with an intramedullary nail. Foot Ankle Int 1999; 20(8):497–500.

19. Yakacki CM, Khalil HM, Dixon SA, et al. Compression forces of internal and external ankle fixation devices with simulated bone resorption. Foot Ankle Int 2010;31(1):76–85.

20. Klos K, Gueorguiev B, Schwieger K, et al. Comparison of calcaneal fixation of a retrograde intramedullary nail with a fixed-angle spiral blade versus a fixed-angle screw. Foot Ankle Int 2009;30(12):1212–8.

21. Santangelo JR, Gilsson RR, Garras DN, et al. Tibiotalocalcaneal arthrodesis: a biomechanical comparison of multiplanar external fixation with intramedullary fixation. Foot Ankle Int 2008;29(9):936–41.

22. Muckley T, Hoffmeier K, Klos K, et al. Angle-stable and compressed angle-stable locking for tibiotalocalcaneal arthrodesis with retrograde intramedullary nails: biomechanical evaluation. J Bone Joint Surg Am 2008;90(3):620–7.

23. Chodos MD, Parks BG, Schon LC, et al. Blade plate compared with locking plate for tibiotalocalcaneal arthrodesis: a cadaver study. Foot Ankle Int 2008;29(2):219–24.

24. O'Neill PJ, Logel KJ, Parks BG, et al. Rigidity comparison of locking plate and intramedullary fixation for tibiotalocalcaneal arthrodesis. Foot Ankle Int 2008;29(6): 581–6.

25. Muckley T, Eichorn S, Hoffmeier K, et al. Biomechanical evaluation of primary stiffness of tibiotalocalcaneal fusion with intramedullary nails. Foot Ankle Int 2007; 28(2):224–31.

26. O'Neill PJ, Parks BG, Walsh R, et al. Biomechanical analysis of screw-augmented intramedullary fixation for tibiotalocalcaneal arthrodesis. Foot Ankle Int 2007; 28(7):804–9.

27. Means KR, Parks BG, Nguyen A, et al. Intramedullary nail fixation with posterior-to-anterior compared to transverse distal screw placement for tibiotalocalcaneal arthrodesis: a biomechanical investigation. Foot Ankle Int 2006;27(12):1137–42.

28. Noonan T, Pinzur M, Paxinos O, et al. Tibiotalocalcaneal arthrodesis with a retrograde intramedullary nail: a biomechanical analysis of the effect of nail length. Foot Ankle Int 2005;26(4):304–8.

29. Bennett GL, Cameron B, Njus G, et al. Tibiotalocalcaneal arthrodesis: a biomechanical assessment of stability. Foot Ankle Int 2005;26(7):530–6.

30. Alfahd U, Roth SE, Stephen D, et al. Biomechanical comparison of intramedullary nail and blade plate fixation for tibiotalocalcaneal arthrodesis. J Orthop Trauma 2005;19(10):703–8.

31. Chiodo CP, Acevedo JI, Sammarco VJ, et al. Intramedullary rod fixation compared with blade-plate-and-screw fixation for tibiotalocalcaneal arthrodesis: a biomechanical investigation. J Bone Joint Surg Am 2003;85(12):2425–8.

32. Berson L, McGarvey WC, Clanton TO. Evaluation of compression in intramedullary hindfoot arthrodesis. Foot Ankle Int 2002;23(11):992–5.

33. Mann MR, Parks BG, Pak SS, et al. Tibiotalocalcaneal arthrodesis: a biomechanical analysis of the rotational stability of the Biomet ankle arthrodesis nail. Foot Ankle Int 2001;22(9):731–3.

34. Greisberg J, Assal M, Flueckiger G, et al. Takedown of ankle fusion and conversion to total ankle replacement. Clin Orthop Relat Res 2004;424:80–8.

35. Gavaskar AS, Chowdary N. Tibiotalocalcaneal arthrodesis using a supracondylar femoral nail for advanced tuberculous arthritis of the ankle. J Orthop Surg (Hong Kong) 2009;17(3):321–4.

36. Nagappa SG, Wood PL. Use of the VersaNnail and anterior ankle arthrotomy to achieve primary tibiotalocalcaneal arthrodesis in rheumatoid arthritis. The Foot 2007;17(3):154–8.

37. Niinimaki TT, Klemola TM, Leppilahti JI. Tibiotalocalcaneal arthrodesis with a compressive retrograde intramedullary nail: a report of 34 consecutive patients. Foot Ankle Int 2007;28(4):431–4.

38. Ahmad J, Pour AE, Raikin SM. The modified use of a proximal humeral locking plate for tibiotalocalcaneal arthrodesis. Foot Ankle Int 2007;28(9):977–83.

39. Boer R, Mader K, Pennig D, et al. Tibiotalocalcaneal arthrodesis using a reamed retrograde locking nail. Clin Orthop Relat Res 2007;463:151–6.

40. Pelton K, Hofer JK, Thordarson DB. Tibiotalocalcaneal arthrodesis using a dynamically locked retrograde intramedullary nail. Foot Ankle Int 2006;27(10):759–63.

41. Goebel M, Gerdesmeyer L, Muckley T, et al. Retrograde intramedullary nailing in tibiotalocalcaneal arthrodesis: a short-term, prospective study. J Foot Ankle Surg 2006;45(2):98–106.

42. Komarasamy B, Best A, Power RA, et al. Outcome following tibiotalocalcaneal fusion with a retrograde intramedullary nail. J Bone Joint Surg Br 2005;88B(Suppl 1):25.

43. Hammett R, Hepple S, Forster B, et al. Tibiotalocalcaneal (Hindfoot) arthrodesis by retrograde intramedullary nailing using a curved locking nail. The results of 52 procedures. Foot Ankle Int 2005;26(10):810–5.

44. Anderson T, Linder L, Rydholm U, et al. Tibio-talocalcaneal arthrodesis as a primary procedure using a retrograde intramedullary nail: a retrospective study of 26 patients with rheumatoid arthritis. Acta Orthop 2005;76(4):580–7.

45. Mendicino RW, Catanzariti AR, Saltrick KR, et al. Tibiotalocalcaneal arthrodesis with retrograde intramedullary nailing. J Foot Ankle Surg 2004;43(2):82–6.

46. Millett PJ, O'Malley MJ, Tolo ET, et al. Tibiotalocalcaneal fusion with a retrograde intramedullary nail: clinical and functional outcomes. Am J Orthop 2002;31(9):531–6.

47. Ebraheim NA, Elgafy H, Stefancin JJ. Intramedullary fibular graft for tibiotalocalcaneal arthrodesis. Clin Orthop Relat Res 2001;385:165–9.

48. Acosta R, Ushiba J, Cracchiolo A. The results of a primary and staged pantalar arthrodesis and tibiotalocalcaneal arthrodesis in adult patients. Foot Ankle Int 2000;21(3):182–94.

49. Chou L, Mann RA, Yaszay B, et al. Tibiotalocalcaneal arthrodesis. Foot Ankle Int 2000;21(10):804–8.

50. Papa JA, Myerson MS. Pantalar and tibiotalocalcaneal arthrodesis for post-traumatic osteoarthrosis of the ankle and hindfoot. J Bone Joint Surg Am 1992;74(7):1042–9.

Management of Severe Deformity Using a Combination of Internal and External Fixation

Rishi Thakral, MBBS, ARFCS, MCh, MSc(Orth Eng), FRCSI (Tr&Orth),
Janet D. Conway, MD*

KEYWORDS

• Deformity • Foot • Ankle • External fixation • Internal fixation

Various pathologic conditions affect the foot and ankle joint and lead to functional failure. Trauma, long-standing inflammatory and crystal arthropathy, infection, neuropathy, osteochondritis, primary arthritis, and congenital foot deformities are a few common conditions seen in day-to-day practice. These conditions eventually change the biomechanics of the joints by altering foot and ankle alignment. Attenuation of the local soft tissue structures, including skin, ligaments, and tendons, causes further deterioration of the function. Painful foot and ankle pathology often leads to limited weight bearing and disuse osteopenia. The resultant deformity with bone and soft tissue abnormalities presents a challenging problem for orthopedic surgeons. Many of these conditions cause severe deformities of the foot and ankle with extreme varus of the distal tibia or hindfoot combined with leg length discrepancies. Also, severe deformities are often accompanied by infection and skin breakdown. These conditions are the most challenging cases for the foot and ankle surgeon, especially when the goal of surgical intervention is to restore the anatomy and achieve a plantigrade, painless, functional foot.[1] This article reviews the surgical techniques used to manage complex foot and ankle deformities, especially the combined techniques of internal and external fixation, and summarizes the results of clinical-based evidence.

Smith & Nephew and Orthofix provided financial support for our institute to host an educational course. Dr Conway has received grants from Medtronic and Synthes.
Rubin Institute for Advanced Orthopedics, International Center for Limb Lengthening, Sinai Hospital of Baltimore, 2401 West Belvedere Avenue, Baltimore, MD 21215, USA
* Corresponding author.
E-mail address: jconway@lifebridgehealth.org

Foot Ankle Clin N Am 16 (2011) 137–163
doi:10.1016/j.fcl.2010.12.002
1083-7515/11/$ – see front matter © 2011 Elsevier Inc. All rights reserved.

foot.theclinics.com

PREOPERATIVE ASSESSMENT

A thorough clinical history includes information about any underlying medical illnesses such as rheumatoid arthritis, diabetes, peripheral vascular disease, and neuromuscular diseases, such as Charcot-Marie-Tooth disease or cerebral palsy. Patients with diabetes who have well-regulated blood sugar levels are less likely to have recurrent infections than those with poorly regulated blood sugar levels.[2] Patients with diminished pulses require a vascular evaluation before formulating a treatment plan. Other critical preoperative information such as steroid use, smoking history, and alcohol use need to be determined. Smoking and steroid use delay wound and bone healing. Alcohol abuse causes osteopenia and also influences a patient's ability to be compliant with postoperative care.[3]

The physical examination should follow the basic rule: look, feel, and move. A thorough physical examination includes the entire lower extremities. Foot and ankle abnormality often compensates for other deformities (eg, fixed subtalar valgus compensating for long-standing genu varum). The symptomatic side is always compared with the contralateral side. Shoes with uneven wear patterns can provide clues about gait. Walking and running gait can be assessed in the office. Running often exaggerates the gait dysfunction and allows the physician to detect otherwise subtle dynamic deformities that are hidden when walking. Any sign of venous stasis, lymphedema, previous surgical scars, healing pattern, ulcers, or skin conditions should be noted. The web spaces between the toes and nails should be inspected closely for hygiene and evidence of any low-grade infection. The foot and ankle region should be palpated to assess the local temperature, points of tenderness, neurovascular status, swelling, and skin scars. Sensation in the distribution of the posterior tibial nerve, superficial peroneal nerve, and sural nerve must be documented. In acute and gradual correction of severe deformities, especially equinus corrections and varus to valgus corrections of the hindfoot, a tarsal tunnel decompression is performed prophylactically. When these decompressions are not done prophylactically, the surgeon must be vigilant to decompress postoperatively at any sign of nerve compromise. A baseline examination is therefore essential and should be well documented to monitor any deterioration during the deformity correction.

Finally, the active and passive ranges of motion should be recorded. These measurements should be obtained in a systemic way, such as proximal to distal. Ankle, subtalar, tarsometatarsal, metatarsophalangeal, and interphalangeal joints should be examined for range of motion and stability. Subtalar joint range of motion is especially important in long-standing deformities. If the subtalar joint is stiff (eg, in severe valgus in the case of compensating for a genu varum), any correction of the genu varum with a high tibial osteotomy would result in a nonplantigrade foot secondary to the fixed subtalar joint valgus. This secondary deformity must be addressed either with the undercorrection of the varus knee, which is not ideal, or a calcaneal osteotomy. Muscle function and power grading of anterior tibialis, toe extensors, peronei, gastrocsoleus complex, tibialis posterior, and toe flexors can be assessed in a systematic clockwise manner. A thorough assessment is tedious but extremely important to document the preoperative function. Any decline in function during deformity correction can then be detected quickly and easily. Clinical photographs should be obtained for a baseline record, whenever possible.

LABORATORY WORKUP

Baseline laboratory work should include complete blood cell count, basic metabolic panel, and levels of C-reactive protein. The laboratory workup of diabetic patients should include levels of blood sugar and glycated hemoglobin. The erythrocyte sedimentation rate (ESR) should be obtained when infection is suspected. ESR is not required routinely but is helpful when the value is more than 70 mm/s, especially when osteomyelitis is suspected.[4]

RADIOLOGY

Radiological evaluation should include the following weight-bearing radiographs:

- Ankle: anteroposterior (AP), lateral, and Saltzman views (to assess hindfoot alignment with tibia) (**Fig. 1**).
- Calcaneus and subtalar joint: Harris axial view.
- Foot: AP, oblique, and lateral views.
- Foot and ankle: stress radiographs of the foot and ankle are helpful when evaluating subtalar joint mobility.
- Limb: a long leg lateral view radiograph should be obtained when proximal sagittal plane deformity is suspected. An erect limb AP view radiograph is useful for frontal plane deformity assessment (**Fig. 2**). Specific deformities affecting the foot and ankle can be caused by genu varum or genu valgum. Leg length discrepancies can also occur after pilon or ankle fractures.

Indium scans are helpful to differentiate infection from Charcot arthropathy, but other nuclear medicine imaging studies are usually not helpful with diagnosis and

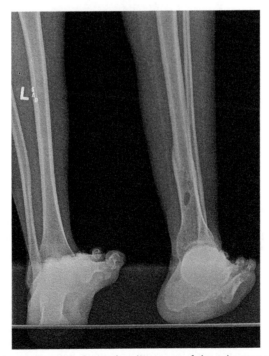

Fig. 1. Saltzman view radiograph shows the alignment of the calcaneus with respect to the distal tibia. In this patient with poliomyelitis, the right calcaneus is in severe varus when compared with the tibia. (*Courtesy of* Rubin Institute for Advanced Orthopedics, Sinai Hospital of Baltimore, copyright 2010; with permission.)

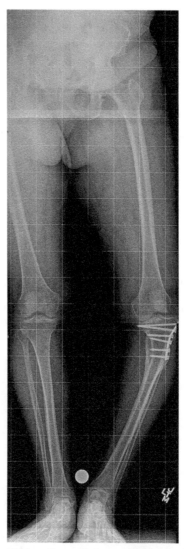

Fig. 2. Weight-bearing erect limb radiograph from the pelvis to the ankles. This patient had severe varus after a malunion of the proximal tibia. Note that the foot is in valgus in order to make it plantigrade. (*Courtesy of* Rubin Institute for Advanced Orthopedics, Sinai Hospital of Baltimore, copyright 2010; with permission.)

surgical planning. A computed tomographic evaluation can delineate bony architecture well, and 3 dimensional reconstruction images can improve the surgeon's understanding of the deformity. Magnetic resonance imaging (MRI) has a role in assessing the extent of osteomyelitis as well as soft tissue infection. This information is useful for planning the worst-case scenario for surgical resection because MRI evaluation is very sensitive to bone marrow edema. Bone marrow edema does not necessarily correlate with bone viability. Bone resection is based on bone viability during surgery. If bone resection is determined only by preoperative MRI evaluation, the surgeon will routinely excise more tissue and bone than necessary, thereby making the reconstruction more difficult and increasing the patient's recovery time.

HARDWARE FOR THE FOOT AND ANKLE: INTERNAL FIXATION VERSUS EXTERNAL FIXATION

Intramedullary rodding is a stable method for fixing severe hindfoot and ankle deformities. The load-bearing ability of the rod allows patients earlier weight bearing after surgery. Severe deformities, however, often make rod insertion a complex task. A common technique used at the authors' center is a fixator-assisted nailing (FAN) approach. The deformity is acutely corrected with an osteotomy, either closing wedge or neutral wedge. The opening wedge osteotomy is reserved for gradual correction. Acute lengthening at the level of the ankle is risky and is associated with poor bone healing, tarsal tunnel symptoms, and skin necrosis. Any prophylactic nerve decompression, such as a peroneal nerve decompression or tarsal tunnel decompression, is done intraoperatively before the osteotomy and deformity correction. To perform FAN, a monolateral fixator is applied to the proximal and distal segments of the deformity (ie, tibia and foot). Care is taken to place the pins out of the path of the intramedullary rod. Ideally, 2 pins are placed proximally and 2 are placed distally (**Fig. 3**). Once the osteotomy is performed, the fixator is used to acutely manipulate the deformity. Once the deformity is completely corrected, the fixator is locked and the rod is inserted without difficulty or fear of undercorrection.

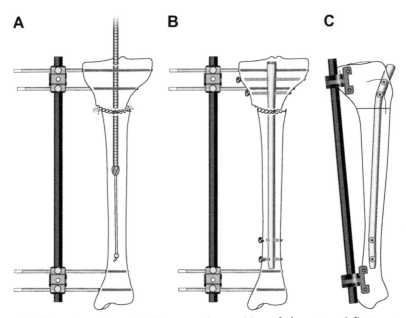

Fig. 3. (*A*) Illustration shows the intraoperative position of the external fixator on the medial side of the tibia, with the temporary fixation pins out of the plane of the intramedullary rod. The osteotomy is performed, and the deformity is acutely corrected and held with the fixator. AP (*B*) and lateral (*C*) view illustrations after intramedullary rod insertion. Note the posterior position of the pins. (*From* Paley D. Principles of deformity correction. Berlin: Springer-Verlag; 2005; with permission.)

Eralp and colleagues[5] recently compared FAN to circular external fixation for correction of angular deformity in patients with rickets. A total of 10 patients (26 limb segments) underwent FAN, and 3 good and 7 excellent bone results were achieved. Seven patients had excellent functional results, 2 had good results, and 1 had a fair result. Two patients who underwent FAN had complications: one had loss of deformity correction and the other had hardware loosening. The circular external fixation group had 9 patients (17 limb segments). Functional and bone results for this group were 7 excellent results and 1 good and 1 fair result. In the circular external fixation group, 66% of patients had pin tract infections and 1 patient experienced premature consolidation of the fibula. No statistically significant differences were observed between the corrections for these 2 groups. The FAN technique is useful, especially for decreasing the prolonged treatment times associated with deformity correction using external fixation only. The 2 contraindications for FAN are the inability to pass a nail through the intramedullary canal of the tibia and/or the hindfoot and the presence of an infection.

In the presence of infection, acute correction of the deformity becomes much more challenging. To consider intramedullary fixation in cases of osteomyelitis, some additional steps are necessary. Intramedullary fixation is an option only if the infection is completely resected. Strict, intraoperative, "clean" and "dirty" procedures need to be followed. Gowns and drapes are replaced and the leg is reprepared after débridement. The dirty instruments for débridement must be contained to 1 Mayo instrument stand, which is discarded after the débridement. After these procedures, an antibiotic-coated intramedullary rod can be safely inserted. Thonse and Conway[6] reported 16 cases of infected ankle and hindfoot fusions treated with antibiotic-coated intramedullary rods. The majority of these cases were successfully treated with 1 surgery (**Fig. 4**).

Just as intramedullary fixation can be used for severe deformities, so can plates, especially locking plates. For the fixator-assisted plating technique, the locking plate construct mimics an external fixator. When the plate is inserted using minimally invasive techniques, blood supply to the bone is preserved because no periosteum stripping is required to seat the hardware next to the bone. The plate is applied close to the mechanical axis of the bone and therefore subjected to less of a bending moment when compared with traditional external fixation.[7] The use of a locking plate allows excellent stability in osteopenic bones.

When internal fixation is not an option, external fixation becomes the treatment of choice. External fixation has great versatility and can be used in the face of acute infection as well as to correct the most severe deformities. The most common external fixation systems used to treat complex deformities are the Ilizarov (Smith & Nephew, Memphis, TN, USA) and the Taylor spatial frame (TSF) (Smith & Nephew, Memphis, TN, USA). Both these frames are circular and are capable of gradual correction through an opening wedge osteotomy. Monolateral frames can also be used for gradual correction. These frames have the advantage of easier application; however, there are fewer options for transfixing the bones of the foot with pins than with wires.

The advantages of external fixation are relatively quick application, minimally invasive approach, less soft tissue disturbance, and the ability to adjust the external fixator at different stages of deformity correction.[8] External fixation allows joint mobility (if desired), allows access to wound care, and is easy to remove after completion of the treatment. The application mode can be static or dynamic, and this adds to the versatility of the treatment approach. External fixation has wide applications for treating various types of fracture patterns, acute and chronic deformities, soft tissue contractures, limb length discrepancies, and segmental bone defects. This type of fixation requires patient motivation and compliance with frequent follow-up visits for

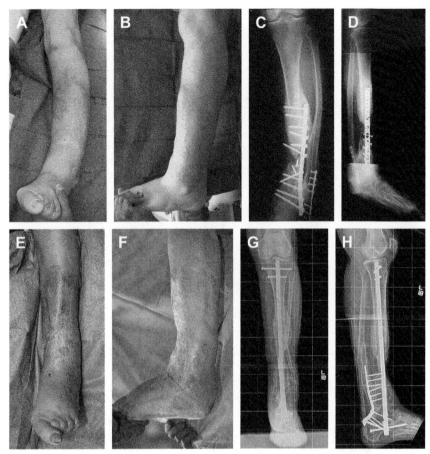

Fig. 4. (*A, B*) Clinical photographs of a patient with a varus ankle and hindfoot combined with infected tibial hardware and osteomyelitis. Preoperative AP (*C*) and lateral (*D*) view radiographs show the varus deformity. Antibiotic-coated intramedullary rod was inserted to treat the infected tibial nonunion and to correct the hindfoot varus simultaneously. (*E, F*) Postoperative photographs show healed skin. Postoperative AP (*G*) and lateral (*H*) view radiographs show varus deformity correction. The ankle nonunion was treated with posterior bone graft. (*Courtesy of* Rubin Institute for Advanced Orthopedics, Sinai Hospital of Baltimore, copyright 2010; with permission.)

assessing the progress of the deformity correction as well as meticulous attention to pin care. Pin site infection, pin loosening, and fracture after removal are just some of the disadvantages.

The 3 main components of the Ilizarov device are as follows: (1) external support (provided by ring and arches), (2) bone fixation (provided by wires and half-pins [hybrid]), and (3) connection (provided by rods, hinges, etc). For frame application, the following systematic approach should be applied. A radiograph should be obtained in a 90° plane (AP and lateral views) to analyze the deformity. The graphic method is used to outline the cross section of bone at its maximum deformity, and the ring size is chosen. The AP deformity is defined on the x-axis, and the lateral deformity is defined on the y-axis of the ordinate system (**Fig. 5**). After connecting the

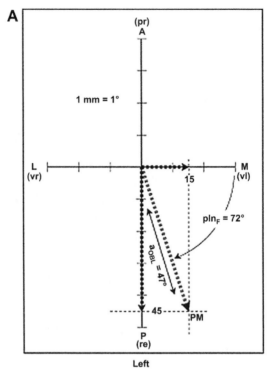

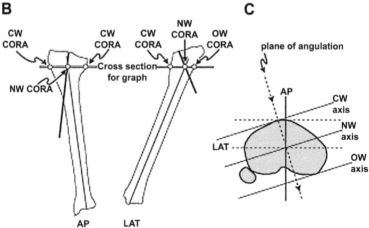

Fig. 5. (*A*) Illustration shows oblique plane deformity planning. The x-axis represents the magnitude of the deformity on the AP view radiograph and the y-axis represents the magnitude of the deformity on the lateral view radiograph. The resultant vector is the magnitude and direction of the oblique deformity. (*B*) Bone schematic shows deformity. (*C*) Cross section of the bone superimposed on the oblique plane deformity graph. A, anterior; a_{OBL}, magnitude of oblique plane angulation; CORA, center of rotation of angulation; CW, closing wedge; L, lateral; LAT, lateral; M, medial; NW, neutral wedge; OW, opening wedge; P, posterior; pln_F, frontal plane of angulation; PM, posteromedial; pr, procurvatum; re, recurvatum; vl, valgus; vr, varus. (*From* Paley D. Principles of deformity correction. Berlin: Springer-Verlag; 2005; with permission.)

points, a rectangular configuration is obtained. A diagonal suspended then defines the true magnitude of the deformity. The angle of inclination is the measure of intersection of the diagonal and the x-axis. The diagonal is the centerpiece, and the hinges are placed in a plane orthogonal to it. Placement of the hinge close to the apex of the deformity determines whether a closing wedge, an opening wedge, or a neutral osteotomy is performed. Opening wedge osteotomy is best tolerated by patients and has the added advantage of restoring bone length. The motor rod is positioned on the concave part of the deformity. Secondary deformity may occur during treatment, which might require replanning the deformity correction. The main limitation of the Ilizarov frame is that it is difficult to correct deformity in 3 planes without major time-consuming frame adjustments in the office.

In the last decade, the principles of deformity correction for foot and ankle have evolved with the availability of the versatile TSF and hydroxyapatite-coated half-pins. The total residual computer software program is especially designed for foot and ankle problems. The TSF is capable of correcting deformity in 3 planes without major frame readjustments. To treat a deformity, the surgeon must determine 3 main parameters: deformity, frame mounting, and structure at risk. Frontal and sagittal deformity parameters are calculated by analyzing the AP and lateral view radiographs. Rotational deformity is assessed clinically. The rings are mounted on the limb orthogonally, matching each fragment of bone. One of the rings is then selected as the reference ring. The reference ring contains the origin fragment and is the nonmoving segment. The other ring moves the corresponding point. After deformity correction, the corresponding point is aligned with the origin. Length is also factored into this calculation because gradual deformity correction is through an opening wedge osteotomy.

The 6 multiplanar struts that are used with rings have hinges built in at both their ends to facilitate deformity correction. Once the deformity parameters, mounting parameters, structure at risk, and strut length/ring size are defined, they are loaded into a software program that prints out a patient schedule. Opening wedge osteotomies are made at the most concave portion of bone, and gradual corrections are performed usually at 1 mm/d. Other considerations for correction speed include the stretch on the most concave portion of skin and soft tissue. If these structures are the most at risk, the speed of correction can be adjusted to allow 1 mm/d (or less) at that soft tissue location.

When considering external fixation for severe deformities, any prophylactic nerve decompression and soft tissue surgery must be completed before the external fixator is applied. It is difficult to perform tarsal tunnel decompression while the patient is in an external fixator. Many studies have reported successful treatment of foot and ankle deformities with gradual correction using external fixation.[2,9–12]

COMBINATION OF INTERNAL AND EXTERNAL FIXATION FOR SEVERE DEFORMITIES OF THE TIBIA, HINDFOOT, AND FOREFOOT

A combination of internal and external fixation is useful in a variety of situations. Patients often do not tolerate prolonged periods of immobilization or non–weight bearing. Also, some patients have demanding jobs or family situations that make it difficult to undergo prolonged treatment for gradual correction and then remain in external fixation for several months until consolidation is achieved. Several techniques can be used that combine internal and external fixation, facilitate decreased external fixation indices, and promote more rapid mobilization. These techniques allow patients to have all the benefits of gradual correction (eg, bone growth, opening wedge osteotomies, minimizing nerve and soft tissue trauma). These techniques include lengthening over a nail (LON), transport over a nail, lengthening and then nailing (LATN), lengthening and then plating (LATP), and gradual correction followed by internal fixation and frame removal.

Other patients who benefit from a combination of internal and external fixation are those who have poor sensation or soft tissue envelopes, which do not allow for extended periods of casting. For patients with diabetes, limited internal fixation is combined with static external fixation, such an ankle arthrodesis. This technique allows full access to the soft tissue envelope. These patients are allowed some weight bearing in the external fixation to increase their mobility.

Lengthening Over a Nail or Transport Over a Nail in the Tibia

Lengthening over a nail follows the same distraction and consolidation phase principles that are used with external fixation. When the distraction phase is finished, the external fixator can be safely removed, and the regenerate bone is allowed to consolidate around the nail. By decreasing the external fixation time, complications such as pin tract infections are eliminated and patients have greater mobility. **Table 1** provides a literature review for lengthening over a nail.

One of the essential concepts when combining internal and external fixation is to keep all external fixation pins and wires away from the internal fixation. In 1997, Paley and colleagues[13] described this LON technique using a cannulated drill over a wire technique to eliminate the rod and pin contact. A 1.8-mm-diameter wire is inserted away from the intramedullary fixation and a C-arm shot is obtained gunsight down the wire. If the wire has adequate bone purchase and has enough clearance for a 6-mm-diameter pin without touching the rod, a 4.8-mm-diameter cannulated drill bit is used to drill over the 1.8-mm-diameter wire. The near cortex is drilled with the cannulated drill and the far cortex is then drilled by exchanging the cannulated drill for a solid one. This step is essential to prevent bone necrosis caused by drilling of the far cortex of hard cortical bone with the flat-tipped cannulated drill. This technique does take time in the operating room and is associated with larger doses of radiation to the surgeon and patient. The trade-off is patient comfort and a diminished risk of intramedullary infection from the external fixation. In the series by Paley and colleagues,[13] the risk of intramedullary infection was 5%. Another essential concept in the LON technique is overreaming the canal to allow the bone segment to move along the rod. Predrilling the osteotomy also allows the reamings to auto bone graft the regenerate. After completion of the distraction phase, the external fixator is removed and the rod is locked with screws. Paley and colleagues,[13] in their series of 32 cases of femoral LON, reported that the mean consolidation index was 1.4 mo/cm for the LON group compared with 1.7 mo/cm for a matched-case external fixation group.

Eralp and colleagues[16] reported 6 cases of distal tibial reconstruction and ankle arthrodesis that were treated using both intramedullary rodding and external fixation for a variety of indications, including osteomyelitis and tumor. Three patients had an average of 5.3 cm of bone loss (range, 2–7 cm), and 4 patients had an average of 5.25 cm of shortening (range, 4–6 cm). The average time in the external fixation was 3.5 months, with a mean external fixation index of 0.57 mo/cm. All patients had excellent bone results, with good functional results in 4 patients and excellent functional results in 2 patients. Three nonoperative complications were reported, including pin tract infection, excessive pain with lengthening, and reflex sympathetic dystrophy. One patient required operative intervention for removal of a painful locking screw.

Kim and colleagues[14] reported 18 tibial cases (13 patients) of LON with insertion of reamed intramedullary nail and application of Ilizarov external fixation. External fixation was used for a mean of 12.5 days. The mean consolidation index was 40.5 d/cm (range, 35.45–51.85 d/cm). The investigators reported no fractures, malalignment, or deep infection with their technique. They reported 2 cases of pin site infection that responded to antibiotic treatment and 3 cases of ankle joint contracture, 1 of which required Achilles tendon lengthening.[14]

Bilen and colleagues[15] described lengthening over a nail with simultaneous correction of tibial deformity. They inserted Schanz pins out of the medullary canal and performed an osteotomy with a multiple drill hole or Gigli saw technique. Deformity correction was performed with uniplanar external fixation assistance, and alignment was confirmed with fluoroscopy. An intramedullary rod was inserted, and the uniplanar external fixator was exchanged with a circular frame. After distraction, the frame was removed and the rod was locked distally for the consolidation phase. In this series of 13 cases, Bilen and colleagues[15] reported an average lengthening of 5.9 cm and a mean bone healing index of 38 d/cm. Complications included equinus contracture (1 patient), delayed healing (2 patients), and compartment syndrome (1 patient). All complications resolved without any residual sequelae.

Wantanabe and colleagues[20] described lengthening over a nail and compared 13 tibial LON cases to 17 standard lengthenings with external fixation. The investigators reported a significantly lower mean external fixation index as well as fewer complications in the LON group. The intraoperative time for the LON group was approximately 1 hour longer when compared with standard intramedullary tibial nailing alone.

Park and colleagues[17] reported tibial LON for short stature in 56 patients. The investigators reported results that were similar to those in the literature, with tibial LON cases having lower external fixation indices and complication rates when compared with traditional external fixation alone. Also, in their series, the patients in the acute treatment who underwent treatment with LON were mobile and were able to function outdoors much better than the traditional external fixation group. However, no difference was reported in the final functional outcome of the 2 groups, with 25% of the patients in each group having occasional difficulties with strenuous activities. Seventy-five percent of the patients in the traditional lengthening group were satisfied with their result compared with 79% of the patients in the LON group.

Pediatric congenital pseudoarthrosis of the tibia (CPT) is a challenge for the orthopedic surgeon and can also be treated successfully using combined external fixation and intramedullary nailing. Mathieu and colleagues[19] treated 10 cases of CPT with combined internal and external fixation. Of the 10 cases, 5 were treated with external fixation and compression and the remaining 5 were treated with segmental bone transport and then compression. The tibiae of 9 of 10 patients were healed at last follow-up without tibial bone grafting. Fibular bone grafting was performed as an intertibiofibular graft in 7 cases, with union in only 5 cases. The average external fixation time was 8.3 months (range 4–13 months). Complications included a superficial pin infection after frame removal that was treated conservatively, 3 ankle valgus deformities, and 3 incomplete lengthenings. One case of deep infection 4 years after external fixator removal necessitated rod removal, with subsequent refracture 2 years later. This patient underwent retreatment with the combined technique and achieved a good result.

Kocaoglu and colleagues[18] published the results of 42 limb segments (35 femora and 7 tibiae) treated with the LON technique. The goal of the study was to determine complications associated with the technique. The mean lengthening was 6.3 cm (range, 2.5–11.5 cm). The mean external fixation index was 18.7 d/cm, and the healing

Table 1
Literature review for the lengthening over nail technique

Authors	Diagnosis	Treatment Method	Number of Cases	Outcome	Complications
Paley et al,[13] 1997	Limb length discrepancy due to various causes (eg, hemihypertrophy, trauma, congenital short femur, achondroplasia, tumor)	LON for femur (Russell-Taylor nail [Smith & Nephew, Memphis, TN, USA] and Ilizarov/Orthofix external fixator)	32 limbs (29 patients)	Radiographic consolidation index: mean, 1.4 mo/cm (range, 0.5–4.5 mo/cm); Excellent results in 23 cases, good in 7, and fair in 2	19 patients had complications. Most common complications: fracture/bending of regenerate bone (n = 4), premature consolidation (n = 4). Minor complications include pin tract infection/loosening, knee contracture (n = 2), peroneal nerve paresis, and delayed union
Kim et al,[14] 2009	Idiopathic dwarfism, trauma, cerebral palsy, hypochondroplasia, neurofibromatosis	LON for tibia (Ilizarov fixator and Dynamic Tibial Nail [DePuyACE, Warsaw, IN, USA] & Metaphyseal/Diaphyseal Nail [Zimmer, Warsaw, IN, USA])	18 limbs (13 patients)	Consolidation index: mean, 40.53 ± 4.92 d/cm (range, 35.45–51.85 d/cm)	8 complications. Most common was ankle contracture (n = 3); minor complications included pin tract infection, paresthesia, and low-back pain
Bilen et al,[15] 2010	Tibial deformity associated with fibular hemimelia, poliomyelitis, constitutional short stature, sequelae of previous lengthening	LON and deformity correction of tibia	13 cases (19 patients)	Mean EFI: 15.8 d/cm (range, 8.9–33.1 d/cm); BHI: mean, 38 d/cm (range, 30–60 d/cm)	4 complications: equinus contracture (n = 1), foot drop/compartment syndrome (n = 1), and delayed union (n = 2)
Eralp et al,[16] 2007	Residual deformity secondary to osteomyelitis, desmoid fibroma, pes calcaneovalgus, poliomyelitis, fibular hemimelia	Combined LON and deformity correction/arthrodesis (Ilizarov external fixation and TriGen intramedullary nail [Smith & Nephew, Memphis, TN, USA])	6 patients	Mean EFI: 0.57 mo/cm. All 6 patients achieved excellent final bone union; excellent function in 2 and good in 4 patients	4 minor complications occurred: pin tract infection, excessive pain, reflex sympathetic dystrophy, and hardware irritation

Study	Indication	Treatment	Patients	Results	Complications
Park et al,[17] 2008	Tibial lengthening for idiopathic short stature	Group A treated with LON with intramedullary nail and Ilizarov external fixator [Smith & Nephew, Memphis, TN, USA]. Group B treated with external fixation (Ilizarov)	44 patients Group A = 56 tibiae Group B = 32 tibiae	Mean preoperative height: 153.7 ± 7.2 cm; Mean postoperative height: 160.1 ± 7.0 cm. Mean gain in tibial length 6.2 cm (20%) Mean gain in tibial length and healing index were the same for both groups	In Group A, 69 complications occurred of which pin tract infection (n = 13), wire/hardware breakage (n = 29), and joint contractures (n = 14) were the most common; others included premature consolidation, neurapraxia, etc
Kocaoglu et al,[18] 2004	Various pathologies including congenital femoral deficiency, fibular hemimelia, infection, trauma, short stature, OI, and rickets	LON and external fixator (Russell-Taylor nail/Orthofix LRS [Orthofix, Richardson, TX, USA]/Hex-Fix external fixator [Smith & Nephew, Memphis, TN, USA])	42 segments (35 femora and 7 tibiae) in 35 patients	Mean lengthening: 6.3 cm (range, 2.5–11.5 cm); Mean EFI: 18.7 d/cm; Lengthening index: 31.2 d/cm	Total 18 complications, most common were nail impingement (33%) and premature consolidation (7.1%); others include pin tract infection, delayed healing, fracture, etc
Mathieu et al,[19] 2008	Congenital pseudoarthrosis of tibia (6 with neurofibromatosis)	Combined external fixation and intramedullary nailing (Ilizarov)	10 patients	9 of 10 achieved union without bone grafting	13 complications, most common were valgus deformity (n = 3) and failure of bone transport (n = 3); others included infection, refracture, and limb length discrepancy

Abbreviations: BHI, bone healing index; EFI, external fixation index; OI, osteogenesis imperfecta.

index was 31.2 d/cm. There were 18 complications (16 limb segments) including screw breakage, screw bending, screw cutout, and pin site infection requiring removal (6 cases). Other complications included premature consolidation of the fibula in tibial LON and 2 equinus contractures requiring percutaneous tendo Achillis lengthening. One case failed to distract secondary to nail impingement at the femoral bow. This complication was treated with nail removal and traditional lengthening. The complication rate was higher in those patients with a lengthening greater than 6 cm or greater than 21.5% of the original bone length.

LATN and LATP

In the LATN technique, the deformity is corrected with external fixation and/or the leg is lengthened and then a second surgical procedure is required to insert the rod and remove the external fixator. This technique is useful for severe deformity corrections that are amenable only to gradual correction with external fixation, yet it has the advantage of allowing the external fixator to be removed before the completion of the consolidation phase. Both the average external fixation time and the complication rates are dramatically reduced with LATN when compared with prolonged external fixation.[21] Another advantage to the LATN technique is that often bone segments are too short for standard intramedullary rods and need to gain adequate length before a rod can be inserted. Also, with large lengthenings, sufficient fixation must remain in the distal segment when the external fixator is removed. If the initial tibial segment is extremely short, traditional lengthening over a nail would not achieve the desired length before the rod would exit the distal segment during the lengthening. The LATN technique also allows removal of the external fixator device during an early phase of treatment, which allows the regenerate bone to consolidate over an intramedullary rod. The other advantage offered by this method is a shorter time to heal. Reaming of the regenerate bone before insertion of the intramedullary rod auto bone grafts the regenerate as well as mechanically stimulates the regenerate. The LATN technique allows the regenerate bone to consolidate more rapidly than the traditional LON technique.[21]

Rozbruch and colleagues[21] in their series of 27 matched-case patients (39 limbs) showed that patients undergoing the LATN technique required 12 weeks of treatment with external fixation. They retrospectively compared 35 tibiae and 4 femora treated by LATN with 31 tibiae and 3 femora that were treated by the classic external fixation method. External fixation was used for 29 weeks in the classic group. The external fixator was applied to the tibia, with the pin and wire fixation placed out of the potential path of the intramedullary rod (**Fig. 6**). The average bone healing index was 0.8 mo/cm for LATN and 1.9 mo/cm in the classic group. For the LATN group, the investigators reported 1 case of sciatic nerve palsy, which resolved without any sequelae, and 1 case of proximal locking screw site infection, which required removal of the hardware and treatment with intravenously administered antibiotics. Two patients required repeat fibular osteotomy for premature consolidation. No fractures occurred, and all bones healed.

Lai and colleagues[22] reported 27 patients who underwent treatment with intramedullary nails after distraction osteogenesis. Intramedullary fixation was done at an average of 3.4 weeks (range 0–15 weeks) after external fixator removal. Bone graft was applied at the rod insertion site in 7 cases. On average, the callus shortening was 0.7 cm (range 0–2.5 cm), with an average healing time of 6.4 months (range, 2–14 months). The union rate in their series was 100%. Complications included 2 cases of distal interlocking screw infection, which resolved on nail removal. Of 26 patients, 17 patients had the rods removed at an average of 26 months after insertion.

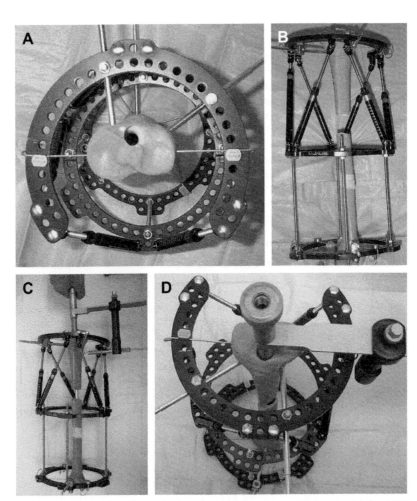

Fig. 6. Photographs of the pin and wire placement on a saw bones model for LATN. (*A*) Bird's-eye view of external fixation away from the intramedullary canal. (*B*) AP view of external fixation after lengthening. (*C*) AP view shows insertion of intramedullary rod around the external fixation. (*D*) Bird's-eye view of rod insertion with external fixation. (*Reprinted from* Springer Science + Business Media: Rozbruch SR, Kleinman D, Fragomen AT, et al. Limb lengthening and then insertion of an intramedullary nail: a case-matched comparison. Clin Orthop Relat Res 2008;466(12):2924; with permission.)

Oh and colleagues[23] describe LATP of 6 tibiae and 4 femora. Diagnoses included infection, Perthes disease, fibular hemimelia, osteosarcoma resection, and tibial dysplasia. The mean external fixation index was 15.1 d/cm, and the average length achieved was 4.0 cm. Nine complications occurred. Oral antibiotics successfully treated four cases of superficial pin tract infections, and physiotherapy was used to resolve four cases of joint stiffness. One patient experienced a fracture of the tibial distraction callus and failure of the locking plate. This fracture healed after re-fixation with a longer locking plate and the addition of more screws. Iobst and Dahl[24] reported on their first 6 patients treated with LATP. The average length achieved was 3.52 cm, with a mean duration of external fixation of 45 days. Complications included a fracture above the plate following a fall and 2 procurvatum deformities of regenerate bone measuring 11° and 18°. No deep infections were reported.

LATP for severe deformity with lengthening is a useful technique to decrease the external fixation times, especially in children. The fixator pins are placed out of the region for the potential plating. The disadvantages of LATP are that the pin sites are stress risers after fixator removal and plating. These sites may lead to fracture with a relatively small amount of trauma because the forces are concentrated there and not at the plate. Also, LATP requires additional skin incisions even when it is inserted atraumatically and in a submuscular/extraperiosteal manner. The last disadvantage, as mentioned in the study by Iobst and Dahl,[24] is the development of procurvatum in 2 cases. This complication is difficult to correct without adjustments to the circular external fixator before plating. Smaller lengthenings can be performed to prevent the progression of the procurvatum with this technique. **Table 2** provides a literature review for LATN and LATP.

Combination Internal and External Fixation Treatment of Acute Trauma

The severely comminuted intra-articular fracture of the distal tibia poses a major challenge for the treating surgeon because of minimal soft tissue envelope coverage. The classic open surgery with internal fixation often has to be delayed to allow the soft tissue edema to resolve. This delay often makes intra-articular reconstruction extremely challenging. External fixation can be applied at an early stage as a definitive treatment as well as to provide good visualization to the traumatized soft tissue envelope. In open fractures, external fixation is mandatory until the risk of infection has subsided. The combined technique of external fixation with minimal internal fixation to restore the articular surface has been successful in preserving soft tissues, obtaining anatomic alignment, and restoring function (**Fig. 7**). **Table 3** provides a literature review for this combination technique for the treatment of acute foot and ankle trauma.

Harris and colleagues[25] retrospectively compared 63 high-energy tibial plafond fractures treated with open reduction and internal fixation (ORIF) with 16 cases treated with limited open reduction and wire external fixation. They reported an equal percentage (2.5%) of wound complications and nonunion in both groups. The rate of posttraumatic arthritis was higher in patients treated with external fixation (68%) when compared with the ORIF group (31.7%). The musculoskeletal function assessment score was higher in the external fixation group (34) than in the ORIF group (20.9). The patients' overall experience was better with ORIF. However, the investigators noted that both techniques can be effective as long as principles of joint restoration, alignment, and stabilization are followed appropriately.

Wyrsch and colleagues[26] conducted a randomized prospective study that compared the ORIF technique with the external fixation technique and observed fewer complications with the latter technique. The investigators observed 15 complications in the ORIF group and 4 in the external fixation group; all complications were related to wound dehiscence and infection. At a minimum follow-up of 2 years, the clinical outcome score was the same for both groups.

Kapoor and colleagues[27] recently reported 17 high-energy pilon fractures treated with indirect reduction of the fracture fragments and capsuloligamentotaxis with an Ilizarov fixator spanning the ankle. The fixator was used to distract the ankle using the calcaneal and proximal tibial rings only. Once the fracture was grossly realigned, tensioned olive wires were inserted into the distal tibial ring to reposition the fracture fragments in anatomic alignment. Other internal fixation hardware (eg, syndesmotic screws) was used as necessary. All cases in their series achieved bony union without

Table 2
Literature review for LATN and LATP techniques

Authors	Diagnosis	Treatment Method	Number of Cases	Outcome	Complications
Rozbruch et al,[21] 2008	Short stature deformity, malunion, nonunion, congenital deformity, poliomyelitis, growth arrest, fibrous dysplasia	LATN for tibia (Ilizarov/ Taylor Spatial Frame [Smith & Nephew, Memphis, TN, USA], EBI/Biomet Monolateral Frame [Biomet, Warsaw, IN, USA])	39 limbs (35 tibiae, 4 femora), 27 patients	Mean EFI: 0.5 mo/cm (range, 0.3–1.1 mo/cm); Mean BHI: 0.8 mo/cm (range, 0.4–1.3 mo/cm)	Most common was joint contracture (n = 17 limbs); other complications were sciatic nerve palsy, skin breakdown, and premature consolidation (n = 2)
Lai et al,[22] 2002	Poliomyelitis, trauma/ bone loss, infection, infected nonunion	LATN (Ilizarov external fixator and locked intramedullary nail)	27 patients	Bone union in all patients at a mean of 6.4 mo (range, 2–14 mo); Mean callus shortening: 0.7 cm (range, 0–2.5 cm)	Common complications: callus fracture (n = 9), docking site nonunion (n = 9), pin tract infection (n = 2)
Oh et al,[23] 2009	LLD due to infection, Perthes disease, fibular hemimelia, osteosarcoma resection, tibial dysplasia	Lengthening (external fixator assisted) and then plating (monorail and circular fixator)	10 patients (6 tibiae, 4 femora)	Mean length: 4.0 cm (range, 3.2–5.5 cm); mean EFI: 15.1 d/cm (range, 13.2–20.5 d/cm); healing index: 48.1 d/cm (range, 41.3 to 55.0 d/cm)	9 complications: pin tract infection (n = 4), joint stiffness (n = 4), and hardware failure (n = 1)
Iobst and Dahl,[24] 2007	Congenital femoral deficiency, post infection LLD, tibial hemimelia, Silver-Russell syndrome, etc	LATP Ilizarov circular fixator/locking compression plate[a]	6 patients (5 femora, 1 tibia)	Solid bony union in all cases (n = 6). Mean EFI: 0.42 mo/cm	3 serious complications: premature consolidation (n = 2), fracture (n = 1); 2 severe complications: residual deformity (n = 2)

Abbreviations: BHI, bone healing index; EFI, external fixation index; LLD, limb length discrepancy.
[a] Manufactured by Synthes Inc, West Chester, PA, USA.

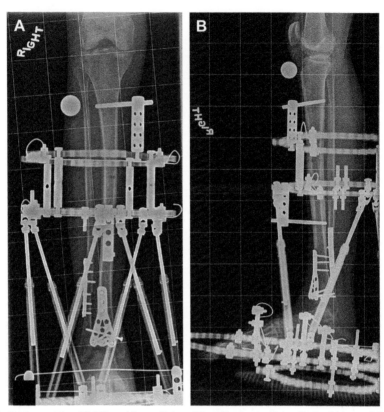

Fig. 7. Postoperative AP (*A*) and lateral view (*B*) radiographs show limited internal fixation to restore the distal tibial articular surface with a spanning external fixator.

wound complications or deep infections from the external fixator. The calcaneal ring was removed at an average of 3.7 weeks postoperatively to allow ankle mobilization. Complications included 9 pin tract infections and 5 malunions, with 1 case undergoing a surgical revision of the external fixator with a good result. Fair, good, and excellent results were observed in 14 of 17 patients.

A similar technique using external fixation combined with limited internal fixation can be performed with calcaneal fractures. Zgonis and colleagues[31] used a calcaneal traction pin with a limited incision on the lateral side of the calcaneus at the level of subtalar joint to elevate the depressed fragments and insert bone graft. The lateral calcaneal wall was then reduced with 2 olive wires inserted from lateral to medial direction. A third wire was placed in the forefoot, and a ring-type fine-wire external apparatus was built. These steps allow weight bearing as early as 1 week after surgery. Paley and Fischgrund[32] also described a limited approach of ligamentotaxis to achieve indirect reduction of the calcaneus using circular external fixation and internal fixation. The investigators first applied an external fixator to realign and distract the heel. They then performed an open reduction and elevated the depressed subtalar fragments. They achieved satisfactory restoration of the anatomy of the joint and the heel in all 6 patients in their series. Four patients had more than 50% of subtalar joint motion, and no patient had any residual heel pain after 2 to 4 years of follow-up.

Combination Internal and External Fixation Treatment of Neuropathic Charcot Ankle and Foot

Charcot foot neuropathy has been known for more then 100 years but still poses a challenge for treatment. Since the mid-1990s, the use of external fixation has gained popularity in treating neuropathic conditions, especially in patients with diabetes. The minimally invasive approach with gradual correction has made it user friendly in complex deformities associated with Charcot foot. Midfoot collapse is the most common in Charcot neuropathy, followed by hindfoot collapse and varus ankle deformity.[33]

It is often difficult to distinguish active infection in patients with acute Charcot arthropathy. Obtaining the C-reactive protein level is somewhat helpful in these cases, but a white blood cell–labeled indium scan is even better. It is important to ensure that there is no active infection with Charcot limb salvage because arthrodeses in these diabetic and neuropathic patients is difficult enough without the additional issue of active infection. Infection eradication is essential before reconstruction.

Midfoot Charcot correction is a staged procedure that consists of correcting the deformity and performing soft tissue releases as necessary. Tendo Achillis lengthening, posterior capsulotomy, flexor hallucis longus and flexor digitorum longus muscle lengthening, and plantar fascial release allow some correction of the deformity. A rigid foot may require an osteotomy. Gradual correction can be achieved by using a butt joint frame (TSF) with tibial and calcaneal components applied orthogonal to the bone axis (**Fig. 8**). Hindfoot correction may be performed acutely after the tendo Achillis lengthening. Once the hindfoot is acutely corrected, U plates are configured around the hindfoot, mounted orthogonal to the tibia. Stirrup wires are applied across the Charcot joint to allow distraction. These wires are fixed to the frame without tension. Struts are then applied, and TSF software is used to program the correction after defining the deformity. To correct the forefoot, a 6 × 6 butt joint frame is applied, which incorporates nontension stirrup wires that are placed close to the osteotomy and are passed through the tarsal bones to allow distraction. Once the hindfoot is corrected and placed into a plantigrade position, the midfoot deformity is unmasked and the degree of apex plantar angulation of the midfoot is often impressive. In the case of severe deformity, it is better to perform an opening wedge gradual osteotomy for correction as opposed to an acute closing wedge osteotomy. If the closing wedge osteotomy is chosen, the foot is dramatically shortened, which makes the foot bulky for shoe wear. Also, wound closure for the acute closing wedge resection is difficult unless performed through a transverse incision.[2] Bone graft may be used as necessary either during osteotomy or during definitive fixation and external fixator removal.

This technique of gradual external fixation followed by internal fixation at the time of external fixator removal has been described by Lamm and Paley[34–36] and Lamm.[37] At the time of fixator removal after gradual forefoot correction, the fixator is prepared and small incisions are made over the midfoot and forefoot joints that need arthrodesis. The joint surfaces are prepared, and bone graft is added as necessary. Guide wires for the large cannulated screws are placed from beneath the metatarsal heads across the midfoot to stabilize the foot position. The frame is removed, and the leg is meticulously reprepared. The large 6.5-mm- or 7.0-mm-diameter partially threaded cannulated screws are then inserted to stabilize the lateral and medial columns of the forefoot. These screws span the length of the forefoot and midfoot and are rigidly fixed into the talus and calcaneus to achieve compression across the arthrodeses. A third central screw is inserted into the second metatarsal and into the hindfoot for stability as well.

Table 3
Literature review for the combination technique for foot and ankle trauma

Authors	Diagnosis	Treatment Method	Number of Cases	Outcome	Complications
Harris et al,[25] 2006	Tibial plafond fractures (21 open fractures): OTA type 43-C3 (n = 43), OTA 43-B1 (n = 5), OTA 43-B2 (n = 4), OTA 43-B3 (n = 2), 43-C1 (n = 15), and OTA type 43-C2 (n = 10)	Limited open reduction (ORIF group and EF group)	79 fractures (76 patients); EF group = 88% open fractures; ORIF group = 44% open fractures	FFI and MFA were higher for EF group with values of 0.40 and 34.0, respectively. For ORIF group, the values were 0.23 and 20.9, respectively.	More complications occurred in the EF group. Posttraumatic arthritis in EF group: 11/16 cases. Malunion rate was higher in ORIF group (3/4 cases). Minor wound complications occurred in both groups
Wyrsh et al,[26] 1996	Tibial plafond fractures; 10 open fractures; Ruedi-Allgower type III (n = 17), type II (n = 14), and type I (n = 8)	Group A = ORIF; group B = external fixation with or without limited internal fixation	Group A = 19 patients; group B = 20 patients	Clinical outcome score (maximum of 140): group A: 61, group B: 73 ($P = .6$); Radiographic score (for available patients): group A: 6 patients had mild, 4 moderate, 4 severe, and 1 no posttraumatic OA; group B: 6 patients developed mild, 8 moderate, 4 severe, and 1 no OA	4 major complications occurred in group B as compared with 15 in group A. Group B: reduced plantar sensation/RSD (n = 1), infection/failure of hardware (n = 1), loss of reduction (n = 1), and pin tract infection (n = 1). Group A: below-knee amputation (n = 3) and other wound complications
Kapoor et al,[27] 2010	Tibial plafond fracture. AO/OTA type 43-B3 (n = 1), type C2 (n = 12), type C3 (n = 4)	Ilizarov external fixation and other hardware as necessary	17 patients	16/17 patients were available for follow-up. All fractures united at a mean of 15.8 wk (range, 13–23 wk). Mean functional ankle score was 79.8 (range, 56–93)	Pin tract infection (n = 9), malunion (n = 4) occurred in 25% of the treated cases

Study	Fracture/Condition	Treatment	Cases	Results	Complications
Ristiniemi et al,[28] 2007	Distal tibia fracture. AO/OTA type A (n = 16), type C (n = 31). 10 open fractures	2-ring hybrid external fixator (Ilizarov)	47 cases	35 cases radiologically united at 20 wk, 12 cases required further surgery for delayed union. RAND 36-item health survey scores for functional assessment were comparable to general population	Pin tract infection (n = 18), and 6 other complications related to hardware (broken wires, penetration of soft tissue or tendons, nerve irritation, nerve injury)
Magnan et al,[29] (2006)	Hindfoot trauma, calcaneal fracture. Sanders type II (n = 15), type III (n = 31), and type IV (n = 8)	Percutaneous reduction and application of Orthofix minifixator	54 cases	Clinical assessment with MFS showed excellent results in 90.7%, fair in 3.7%, and poor in 5.6%; CT scan (SAVE) showed excellent results in 44.4%, good in 46.3%, fair in 5.6%, and poor in 3.7% of the cases; Böhler calcaneal angle was restored from a mean of 6.98° preop to 21.94° postop	18.5% transient osteoporosis (n = 10), 5.6% skin infection (n = 3), 5.6% thalamic displacement upon weight bearing (n = 3)
Chandran et al,[30] 2006	Severe midfoot trauma, open wounds to severe degloving injuries	Biplanar external fixator and K-wires	11 patients	All fractures united at 1-year follow-up	Flatfoot (n = 3), cavus foot (n = 4), malunion (n = 4), ankylosis (n = 1). All had stiffness of subtalar and forefoot joints

Abbreviations: AO, Association for Osteosynthesis; CT, computed tomography; EF, external fixation; FFI, foot function index; K-wire, Kirschner wire; MFA, musculoskeletal function assessment score; MFS, Maryland foot score; OA, osteoarthritis; ORIF, open reduction and internal fixation; OTA, Orthopaedic Trauma Association; preop, preoperative; postop, postoperative; RSD, reflex sympathetic dystrophy; SAVE, score analysis of Verona.

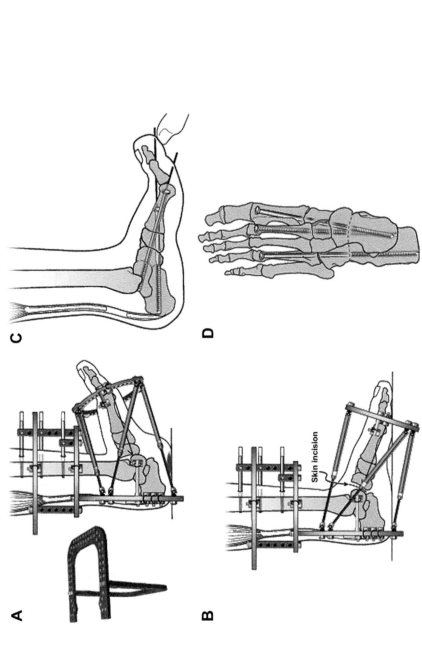

Fig. 8. (*A*) TSF butt joint frame construct. (*B*) Position of the TSF after gradual correction of midfoot Charcot deformity. Lateral (*C*) and AP (*D*) view illustrations of the intramedullary fixation after external fixator removal. (*Courtesy of* Rubin Institute for Advanced Orthopedics, Sinai Hospital of Baltimore, copyright 2010; with permission.)

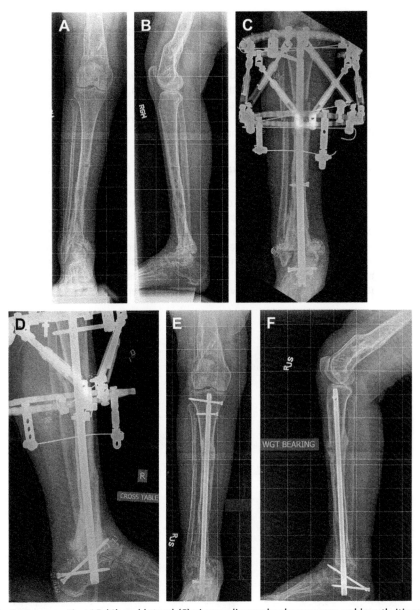

Fig. 9. Preoperative AP (*A*) and lateral (*B*) view radiographs show severe ankle arthritis and a tibial leg length discrepancy. Postoperative AP (*C*) and lateral (*D*) view radiographs show external fixation and a long, custom, ankle and hindfoot fusion rod. Note the proximal tibial osteotomy for bone transport and the custom interlocking hole in the midshaft of the tibia to keep the ankle arthrodesis from distracting while lengthening the tibia. Postoperative AP (*E*) and lateral (*F*) view radiographs with a well-healed ankle arthrodesis and tibial regenerate at the end of treatment. WGT bearing, weight bearing. (*Courtesy of* Rubin Institute for Advanced Orthopedics, Sinai Hospital of Baltimore, copyright 2010; with permission.)

A non–weight-bearing cast is applied for 2 to 3 months, with progression to full weight bearing. Custom orthotics are made once the patient progresses to normal shoe wear. The total treatment time is approximately 4 to 5 months, with 2 months for gradual correction in the external fixator. Lamm and colleagues[11] reported on a series of 11 limbs in 8 patients. Postoperatively, statistically significant improvements were noted in the calcaneal pitch, AP talar–first metatarsal angle, and the lateral talar–first metatarsal angle. The investigators observed no deep infections, hardware failures, or recurrent ulcerations at an average follow-up of 22 months. No patients underwent amputation.

Combination Internal and External Fixation Treatment of Limb Salvage Ankle Arthrodesis

Very few articles have been published on using a combination of internal and external fixation to treat failed ankle arthrodeses and other severe foot and ankle deformities. Mendicino and colleagues[38] published a case report using a 2-stage approach: insertion of an intramedullary antibiotic-coated guide rod to eradicate the intramedullary infection and then revision ankle arthrodesis with a circular external fixator. Chen and colleagues[39] reported 12 cases of ankle arthrodesis using a combination of intramedullary nails and external fixation. All cases had preoperative osteomyelitis treated

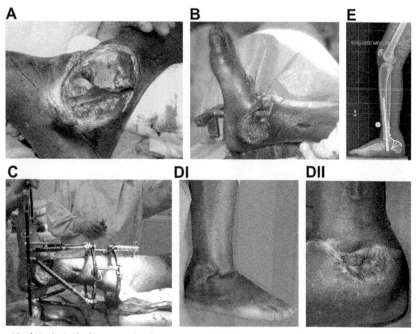

Fig. 10. (*A*) Clinical photograph of a 50-year-old diabetic man with severe open ankle injury and massive soft tissue loss. Clinical postoperative photographs obtained after antibiotic-coated rod insertion (*B*) and external fixator application to gradually compress an 8-cm gap of bone and soft tissue (*C*). (*D*) Clinical photographs (I and II) show the stable and closed soft tissue envelope after split thickness skin grafting to the medial and lateral sides. (*E*) Postoperative lateral view radiograph shows the locked rod after external fixator removal and subsequent posterior bone grafting to ankle nonunion. (*Courtesy of* Rubin Institute for Advanced Orthopedics, Sinai Hospital of Baltimore, copyright 2010; with permission.)

with radical resection followed by segmental bone transport. All cases were ambulatory and without infection at the latest follow-up. However, 4 cases had rod removal for infection during treatment, which resolved with removal and antibiotics. At the authors' center, the combined technique is used when possible. **Figs. 9** and **10** show 2 cases of limb salvage ankle arthrodesis with internal and external fixation.

SUMMARY

The goals of treatment should be to achieve a stable, functional, and pain-free plantigrade foot. In severe deformities of the foot and ankle associated with bone loss and limb length discrepancy, the combined techniques of internal and external fixation are effective in decreasing the external fixation time and increasing the patient's comfort. The surgeon and the patient, however, must be aware of the slight increased risk of infection with the internal fixation in these cases. In these complex problems, the benefits of decreased fixator time are worth the risk, especially when the patients are unable to comply with prolonged treatment times. As this combined technique becomes more popular with surgeons as well as patients, more studies will need to be published that critically evaluate the results.

ACKNOWLEDGMENTS

The authors would like to thank the following people for their invaluable assistance with the manuscript: Dr Bradley M. Lamm, Dr S. Robert Rozbruch, Alvien Lee, Joy Marlowe, MA, and Amanda Chase, MA.

REFERENCES

1. Wardak M, Wardak E, Goel A. Calcanisation of tibia using Ilizarov fixator in crush injuries of hindfoot: a new method. Int Orthop 2008;32:779–84.
2. Conway JD. Charcot salvage of the foot and ankle using external fixation. Foot Ankle Clin 2008;13(1):157–73, vii.
3. Alvisa-Negrín J, González-Reimers E, Santolaria-Fernández F, et al. Osteopenia in alcoholics: effect of alcohol abstinence. Alcohol Alcohol 2009;44(5):468–75.
4. Jolly GP, Zgonis T, Polyzois V. External fixation in the management of Charcot neuroarthropathy. Clin Podiatr Med Surg 2003;20(4):741–56.
5. Eralp L, Kocaoglu M, Toker B, et al. Comparison of fixator-assisted nailing versus circular external fixator for bone realignment of lower extremity angular deformities in rickets disease. Arch Orthop Trauma Surg 2010. [Epub ahead of print].
6. Thonse R, Conway JD. Antibiotic cement-coated nails for the treatment of infected nonunions and segmental bone defects. J Bone Joint Surg Am 2008; 90(Suppl 4):163–74.
7. Haidukewych GJ. Innovations in locking plate technology. J Am Acad Orthop Surg 2004;12(4):205–12.
8. Fragomen AT, Rozbruch SR. The mechanics of external fixation. HSS J 2007;3(1): 13–29.
9. Zgonis T, Roukis TS, Lamm BM. Charcot foot and ankle reconstruction: current thinking and surgical approaches. Clin Podiatr Med Surg 2007;24(3):505–17, ix.
10. Zgonis T, Stapleton JJ, Roukis TS. Use of circular external fixation for combined subtalar joint fusion and ankle distraction. Clin Podiatr Med Surg 2008;25(4): 745–53, xi.

11. Lamm BM, Gottlieb HD, Paley D. A two-stage percutaneous approach to Charcot diabetic foot reconstruction. J Foot Ankle Surg 2010;49(6):517–22.

12. Lamm BM, Standard SC, Galley IJ, et al. External fixation for the foot and ankle in children. Clin Podiatr Med Surg 2006;23(1):137–66, ix.

13. Paley D, Herzenberg JE, Paremain G, et al. Femoral lengthening over an intramedullary nail. A matched-case comparison with Ilizarov femoral lengthening. J Bone Joint Surg Am 1997;79(10):1464–80.

14. Kim H, Lee SK, Kim KJ, et al. Tibial lengthening using a reamed type intramedullary nail and an Ilizarov external fixator. Int Orthop 2009;33(3):835–41.

15. Bilen FE, Kocaoglu M, Eralp L, et al. Fixator-assisted nailing and consecutive lengthening over an intramedullary nail for the correction of tibial deformity. J Bone Joint Surg Br 2010;92(1):146–52.

16. Eralp L, Kocaoglu M, Yusof NM, et al. Distal tibial reconstruction with use of a circular external fixator and an intramedullary nail. The combined technique. J Bone Joint Surg Am 2007;89(10):2218–24.

17. Park HW, Yang KH, Lee KS, et al. Tibial lengthening over an intramedullary nail with use of the Ilizarov external fixator for idiopathic short stature. J Bone Joint Surg Am 2008;90(9):1970–8.

18. Kocaoglu M, Eralp L, Kilicoglu O, et al. Complications encountered during lengthening over an intramedullary nail. J Bone Joint Surg Am 2004;86(11):2406–11.

19. Mathieu L, Vialle R, Thevenin-Lemoine C, et al. Association of Ilizarov's technique and intramedullary rodding in the treatment of congenital pseudarthrosis of the tibia. J Child Orthop 2008;2(6):449–55.

20. Watanabe K, Tsuchiya H, Sakurakichi K, et al. Tibial lengthening over an intramedullary nail. J Orthop Sci 2005;10(5):480–5.

21. Rozbruch SR, Kleinman D, Fragomen AT, et al. Limb lengthening and then insertion of an intramedullary nail: a case-matched comparison. Clin Orthop Relat Res 2008;466(12):2923–32.

22. Lai KA, Lin CJ, Chen JH. Application of locked intramedullary nails in the treatment of complications after distraction osteogenesis. J Bone Joint Surg Br 2002;84(8):1145–9.

23. Oh CW, Song HR, Kim JW, et al. Limb lengthening with a submuscular locking plate. J Bone Joint Surg Br 2009;91(10):1394–9.

24. Iobst CA, Dahl MT. Limb lengthening with submuscular plate stabilization: a case series and description of the technique. J Pediatr Orthop 2007;27(5):504–9.

25. Harris AM, Patterson BM, Sontich JK, et al. Results and outcomes after operative treatment of high-energy tibial plafond fractures. Foot Ankle Int 2006;27(4):256–65.

26. Wyrsch B, McFerran MA, McAndrew M, et al. Operative treatment of fractures of the tibial plafond. A randomized, prospective study. J Bone Joint Surg Am 1996;78(11):1646–57.

27. Kapoor SK, Kataria H, Patra SR, et al. Capsuloligamentotaxis and definitive fixation by an ankle-spanning Ilizarov fixator in high-energy pilon fractures. J Bone Joint Surg Br 2010;92(8):1100–6.

28. Ristiniemi J, Flinkkilä T, Hyvönen P, et al. Two-ring hybrid external fixation of distal tibial fractures: a review of 47 cases. J Trauma 2007;62(1):174–83.

29. Magnan B, Bortolazzi R, Marangon A, et al. External fixation for displaced intra-articular fractures of the calcaneum. J Bone Joint Surg Br 2006;88(11):1474–9.

30. Chandran P, Puttaswamaiah R, Dhillon MS, et al. Management of complex open fracture injuries of the midfoot with external fixation. J Foot Ankle Surg 2006;45(5):308–15.

31. Zgonis T, Roukis TS, Polyzois VD. The use of Ilizarov technique and other types of external fixation for the treatment of intra-articular calcaneal fractures. Clin Podiatr Med Surg 2006;23(2):343–53, vi–vii.

32. Paley D, Fischgrund J. Open reduction and circular external fixation of intraarticular calcaneal fractures. Clin Orthop Relat Res 1993;290:125–31.

33. Sticha RS, Frascone ST, Wertheimer SJ. Major arthrodeses in patients with neuropathic arthropathy. J Foot Ankle Surg 1996;35(6):560–6.

34. Lamm BM, Paley D. Minimally invasive realignment surgery for the Charcot foot. In: Scuderi GR, Tria AJ, editors. Minimally invasive surgery in orthopedics. New York: Springer; 2009. p. 443–8.

35. Lamm BM, Paley D. Reduction of neuropathic foot deformity with gradual external fixation distraction and midfoot fusion. In: Frykberg RG, editor. The diabetic Charcot foot: principles and management. Brooklandville (MD): Data Trace Publishing Company; 2009. p. 195–208.

36. Lamm BM, Paley D. Minimally invasive realignment surgery of the Charcot foot. In: Wiesel SW, editor-in-chief, Operative techniques in orthopaedic surgery, vol. 4. Philadelphia: Lippincott Williams & Wilkins; 2011. p. 3809–13.

37. Lamm BM. Surgical reconstruction and stepwise approach to acute Charcot neuroarthropathy. In: Zgonis T, editor. Surgical reconstruction of the diabetic foot and ankle. Philadelphia: Lippincott Williams & Wilkins; 2009. p. 223–9.

38. Mendicino RW, Bowers CA, Catanzariti AR. Antibiotic-coated intramedullary rod. J Foot Ankle Surg 2009;48(2):104–10.

39. Chen CM, Su AW, Chiu FY, et al. A surgical protocol of ankle arthrodesis with combined Ilizarov's distraction-compression osteogenesis and locked nailing for osteomyelitis around the ankle joint. J Trauma 2010;69(3):660–5.

Hindfoot Arthrodesis for Management of Bone Loss Following Calcaneus Fractures and Nonunions

Andy P. Molloy, FRCS (Tr&Orth)*, Stephen J. Lipscombe, MRCS

KEYWORDS

• Calcaneus • Fracture • Malunion • Nonunion • Arthrodesis

Calcaneal fractures are the most common of tarsal bone fractures accounting for 2% of all fractures.[1] The most common cause for these fractures is either a fall from height or motor vehicle accidents. Because of the forces necessary to produce these fractures, patients with calcaneal fractures can have associated spinal fractures and other peripheral injuries. The huge forces involved in the cause of these fractures cause compression, bone loss, and therefore displacement. These results can lead to widening of the heel, loss of heel height, and large amounts of displacement of the articular surfaces. Introduction of modern internal fixation methods has decreased the incidence of necessity of hindfoot arthrodesis for management of bone loss and nonunion of calcaneal fractures; yet, unfortunately, it is still prevalent.

These disabling injuries have a huge symptomatic effect on patients. They also often have a huge economic impact because most fractures occur in adults in their economic prime, who are frequently industrial workers.

There is another subgroup of patients who sustain massive calcaneal bone loss. These are patients who sustain open injuries. There are 2 common causes for these severe injuries. The first is through high-force crush injuries, in which the injuries are often complicated by massive contamination. The second cause is blast injuries that can occur both in the industrial setting and in those who are gallantly serving their country in military.

The authors have nothing to disclose.
Department of Orthopaedics and Trauma, University Hospital Aintree, Lower Lane, Liverpool, L9 7AL, United Kingdom
* Corresponding author.
E-mail address: orthoblue@aol.com

Foot Ankle Clin N Am 16 (2011) 165–179
doi:10.1016/j.fcl.2010.12.008
foot.theclinics.com

CLOSED INJURIES
Overview of Treatment of Acute Fractures

Dilemma still exists as to whether operative fixation provides better functional outcome than nonoperative management, which avoids the complications of wound infection, skin breakdown, and nerve injury.

Painful subtalar arthrosis is a major sequela of calcaneal fracture.[2] This situation is not true in all cases and many patients can function well and return to employment; however, over the course of 20 years, function does deteriorate correlating with arthroses as determined by computed tomographic (CT) scanning. Whether operative reduction and fixation can avoid such deterioration was refuted in the study by Ibrahim and colleagues,[3] with a 15-year follow-up period following randomization to operative and nonoperative management. They suggested that there was no difference in functional outcome between operative and nonoperative groups. Nonoperative management consisted of elevation and compression to control swelling initially, then early mobilization of the foot as pain allowed but non–weight bearing for up to 8 weeks. Operative management consisted of an open lateral approach to the calcaneus, reduction and fixation with K wires, followed by cast immobilization and non–weight bearing for 8 weeks. At 15-year follow-up, no patients had undergone subtalar fusion or were listed for such a procedure.

The study by Parmar and colleagues[4] produced similar results. Undisplaced fractures resulted in excellent outcome, regardless of treatment. Displaced fractures treated nonoperatively had reasonable function, which operative fixation failed to improve significantly.

These studies would seem to provide the answer to the management of calcaneal fractures. However, there have been many advances in approach and implants available since these studies were published. Arthroses of the subtalar joint occur at some point following the injury, although with poor correlation to the degree of functional impairment, so that operative fixation fails to prevent this outcome. Meta-analyses performed by Randle and colleagues[5] and Bajammal and colleagues[6] concluded that the evidence for operative fixation remained weak, with a trend toward better outcomes, but study numbers tended to be small and concluded that there was insufficient evidence to confirm that operative fixation is the best option, although arthrodesis rates were noted to be lower in the fixation group. Such is the complexity of the articular facets of the calcaneus that open reduction, even supplemented by intraoperative fluoroscopy, fails to reconstruct the articular surface.[7]

Perhaps, of greatest note from the meta-analyses is the variation between the studies. Variation exists in surgical techniques and the assessment of outcomes. If the outcome is a painful degenerative arthrosis, it is commonly measured as those patients are progressing to subtalar arthrodesis. It might be considered that accurate anatomic reduction of the articular surface of the calcaneus would improve such scores.

Medial approaches have been used in some studies to achieve reduction, but Eastwood and colleagues[8,9] examined the fracture configurations using CT scan and noted that instrumentation and reduction of the lateral wall fragment was almost always necessary and that such exposure allows reduction of such fragments onto the sustentaculum medially. The advantage of the lateral approach is the excellent exposure of the tuberosity, posterior facet, lateral wall, and calcaneocuboid articulation. Schepers and colleagues[10] have recently described closed reduction and percutaneous fixation of severely comminuted fractures of the os calcis. They reported satisfactory reduction and function up to 1 year, although some patients subsequently underwent subtalar arthrodesis. Zwipp and colleagues[11] performed both a medial approach and then a lateral approach for fracture fixation and noted improved outcome.

Earlier studies tended to use K-wire or screw fixation to maintain the reduced articular surface. The Cochrane review of Bridgman and colleagues[12] in 2000 was withdrawn in 2008 because it was thought to be out of date. The suggestion was that although reduction was achieved, the stability of fixation was inadequate with wire and screw fixation, especially in crushed cancellous bone. Leung and colleagues[13] supported operative plate fixation of intra-articular fractures. The groups were slightly skewed with a smaller group of patients undergoing nonoperative management, and there was no clear indication as to what this approach consisted of. Patient outcome measures were determined by an obscure scoring system that demonstrated significant differences between pain and function, favoring operative fixation, with 3 nonoperative patients requiring subtalar arthrodesis. Follow-up period was limited to only 3 years. Allmacher and colleagues[2] have already suggested that symptomatic arthroses can take more than 10 years to develop.

Loucks and Buckley[14] and Crosby and Fitzgibbons[15] have noted that the correlation between functional outcome and the Bohler angle depends on the angle at presentation rather than on subsequent management. Although operative treatment improved the angle, there was no significant difference in the functional scoring of these patients compared with those managed nonoperatively. This result suggests that the high-energy injury to the soft tissue and articular surface, which obliterates the Bohler angle, has a poor prognosis, regardless of operative management, restoration, and rigid fixation. Paul and colleagues[16] completed a 6.5-year follow-up of patients treated either nonoperatively or operatively. They determined that a Bolher's angle of less than 10 degrees was associated with poor outcome if treated operatively but even worse if treated non-operatively, with increasing levels of pain and subsequent subtalar arthrodesis. Groups with a Bohler angle greater than 10° that underwent fixation functioned well. Patients with undisplaced fractures managed nonoperatively performed best. Surgery for more-simple fracture patterns, which could be reduced and managed with operative fixation, has been supported by other investigators.[17–19] Csizy and colleagues[20] examined specifically those patients who underwent delayed subtalar arthrodesis following calcaneal fracture. They identified that the initial Bohler angle was the most significant factor in these patients. According to Bajammal and colleagues,[6] heavy manual workers and increasing severity of fracture pattern were also important factors. A greater number of patients managed nonoperatively also underwent delayed fusion.[20]

There can be minor superficial wound problems (8%–16%), with some progressing to deep infection requiring debridement and occasional fasciocutaneous flap treatment (1.9%–4%) noted with lateral plating.[21–24] These studies also report prominent metalwork, inadequate fixation with penetration of the joint surface, and sural nerve injury.

Complications of wound infection and breakdown should be considered, but the pain from a grossly incongruent joint and the resultant subtalar stiffness may, however, be managed better with meticulous reduction and stabilization. O'Brien and colleagues[25] suggest that in younger adults, accurate reduction of the fracture results in higher gait satisfaction scores than those treated nonoperatively. The function of the hindfoot is significantly improved if the calcaneus is restored to its normal shape, allowing a more normal gait pattern, which correlated with improved functional scores.[26,27]

Stabilization with external fixators using closed and mini-open reduction techniques has also been described.[28,29] The results were excellent in most patients. Superficial pin infection was a minor problem. Emara and Allam[30] have used the Ilizarov technique for the management of fractures with poor skin condition, noting the main complication of wound infection and dehiscence following open reduction and internal fixation. The frame produced similar functional results to those treated with standard lateral approach and plate fixation. Wound infection did occur in the plate fixation group, with 1 patient requiring debridement. Two pin-site infections were noted in the frame group. The compliance with such frames, quality of reduction, and stability of the constructs have also yet to be proved.

Schepers and colleagues[10] have previously described the use of a distraction system and K-wire fixation of calcaneal fractures using percutaneous techniques. Although such techniques can be useful in open injuries or with tenuous soft tissues, there are concerns regarding the quality of reduction and the stability of fixation achievable with these techniques.[31]

Functional results following calcaneal fracture have been examined by Tufescu and Buckley.[32] They have described that return to work is quicker following operative fixation in all workers, with a mean duration of 87 days, although heavy laborers took 171 days to return. This mean duration was shorter than that in patients treated nonoperatively. Heavy manual laborers failed to return to their preinjury work intensity.

In a small study, O'Farrell and colleagues[33] concluded that more patients returned to work and were able to walk further than patients treated nonoperatively. Additionally, shoe wear was more difficult for the varus malunion, although Kundel and colleagues'[34] study outcome at 5 years found that only return to work was influenced by operative fixation, with no significant differences in pain or shoe wear.

Given the uncertainty of operative results for the most severely displaced fractures and the complications of nonoperative management, with pain, gait disturbance, and lateral exostectomy for prominent malunion, can primary subtalar fusion provide better functional results than attempted reconstruction, which then fails and requires arthrodesis?[35,36] Reddy and colleagues[37] report that reconstruction should still be attempted, given the disability following subtalar arthrodesis. Flemister and colleagues[38] also suggested that although primary subtalar arthrodesis can be used for the management of calcaneal fractures, arthrodesis following fixation of calcaneal fracture can be achieved with equally satisfactory results with union rates of 96%. Techniques have been described including a sliding calcaneal osteotomy with primary subtalar fusion[39] and an in situ arthrodesis with distraction bone grafting.[40]

Etiology, Classification, and Deformity of Malunions

Calcaneal malunions with massive bone loss have become less prevalent over the past 3 decades because of the popularization of modern methods of internal fixation of acute fractures. Although hindfoot arthrodesis may be necessary, the normal overall architecture should have been restored. However, as outlined in the previous section, there are still many advocates of nonoperative treatment of displaced intra-articular fractures. There are also certain subgroups of patients who are possibly not suitable for primary internal fixation (eg, patients with severe peripheral vascular disease, elderly diabetic patients, drug-dependent patients). However, there is also a subgroup of patients who have been initially treated operatively and have developed large intra-articular cavities because of loss of reduction caused by poor stabilization of the fracture.

Stephens and Sanders[41] reported a classification system for calcaneal malunions, which included 3 types. Type 1 malunions have a lateral wall exostosis with normal hindfoot alignment. Type 2 malunions have a lateral wall exostosis, subtalar arthrosis, and hindfoot malalignment of less than 10°. Type 3 malunions feature the same abnormalities as type 2 but have greater than 10° of malalignment.

The malalignment is usually a varus deformity of the calcaneal body. It may also include superior translation of the calcaneal tuberosity. The lateral wall exostosis is formed by the united lateral wall blow out and by the superolateral translation. The exostosis can cause subfibular impingement and peroneal pathology including tears of the peroneus brevis and subluxation or dislocation of both peronei. The exostosis, varus deformity, and foreshortening of the heel also have the effect of widening the heel.

Bone loss, caused by crushing from the force of the initial injury, causes residual articular incongruity. The obvious effect of this incongruity is ensuing subtalar posttraumatic arthritis. However, the anterior extension of the primary fracture line can cause incongruity, and thereby posttraumatic arthritis, of the calcaneocuboid joint. If the bone loss is more severe, then there are additional effects on hindfoot and ankle function. Even if there is a superiorly translated malunion of the calcaneal tuberosity, the bone loss causes an overall loss in bone height. This loss can shorten the gastro-soleus lever arm and thereby reduces the push-off strength.[42,43] The talus, obviously, settles into the defect in the calcaneal articulation of the subtalar joint. This effect alters the talocalcaneal angle and the talar declination angle. Both these deformities significantly alter hindfoot movements and if left untreated, cause posttraumatic arthritis in all 3 hindfoot joints. The alteration in talar declination angle may cause ankle stiffness (**Fig. 1**). The anterior impingement becomes more pronounced with more pronounced alterations in the talar declination angle, which can even be reversed with the most severe defects.

Nonunion is a rarely reported complication of calcaneal fractures (**Fig. 2**). Zwipp and colleagues[11] reported a nonunion rate of 1.3% in a series of 157 fractures treated with open reduction internal fixation. There are 2 main reasons for this result. First, the calcaneus is mainly composed of cancellous bone. Second, the extensile L-shaped lateral incision is specifically designed to lessen damage to the osseous (and cutaneous) blood supply. Smoking, diabetes, and open fractures have all been demonstrated to be independent risk factors for wound complications in the initial operative treatment of calcaneal fractures,[44] which is also true for osseous complications. However, in the series reported by Molloy and colleagues,[45] 86% of the cases had poor quality initial reduction and hardware placement and 20% had chronic deep infection.

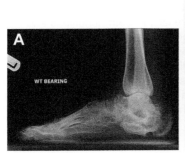
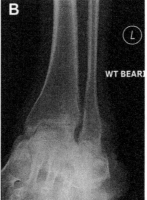

Fig. 1. Radiographs of type 3 malunion. (*A*) Lateral weight-bearing foot. (*B*) Anteroposterior weight-bearing ankle.

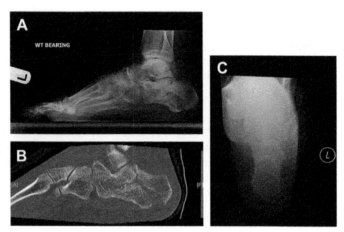

Fig. 2. Nonunion of the body of the calcaneus. (*A*) Lateral weight-bearing radiograph of foot. (*B*) Sagittal CT view. (*C*) Axial radiograph of calcaneus.

Assessment of calcaneal malunions and nonunions

A thorough history and examination are obviously essential. If a nonunion is present, then any potential history of infection should be sought out. Range of motion of the hindfoot and ankle should be carefully assessed and compared with the contralateral side. The subtalar, calcaneocuboid, talonavicular, and ankle joints should all be assessed for any of the stigmata of posttraumatic arthritis. The appearance and plane (as well as timing) of incisions should be noted. The relative length of the heel and the prominence of the calcaneal tuberosity should be compared with the contralateral side. The extent of the lateral wall exostosis should be assessed together with the presence of any subfibular impingement and peroneal pathology (tears, subluxation, or dislocation).

Standard weight-bearing ankle and foot radiographs should be taken. Assessment of the Bohler angle, the crucial angle of Gissane, talar declination angle, talocalcaneal height, and talocalcaneal angle provides valuable information on the degree of bone loss (**Fig. 3**). Calcaneal axial and Coby view radiographs provide further information on calcaneal deformity. Lateral weight-bearing forced dorsiflexion and plantar-flexion views delineate any anterior tibiotalar impingement. All of the aforementioned views also demonstrate the presence of arthritis. Comparative views of the other foot should be taken as necessary.

A CT scan is essential if there is any suspicion of a nonunion. The scan image delineates the planes of the nonunion, so that an accurate preoperative plan can be made. A 3-dimensional reconstruction can be useful in both nonunions and malunions for obtaining a better judgment on the magnitude and plane of deformity. If there is any potential history of low-grade infection, then further investigation is warranted. Magnetic resonance imaging with gadolinium is both sensitive and specific for infection but is of more limited value if stainless steel implants are present. In this scenario, a dual isotope scan is the investigation of choice. However, the specificity is reduced if there is less than 1 year duration after the index procedure.

Treatment of malunions

Treatment of type 1 malunions (lateral wall exostosis alone) simply involves a lateral wall exostectomy (and treatment of any peroneal pathology present). The procedure

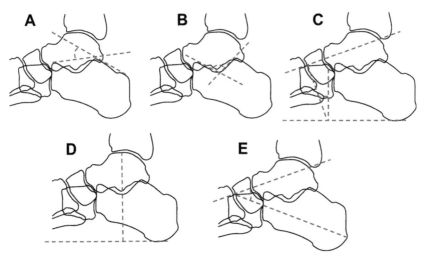

Fig. 3. Radiographic angles for assessment of calcaneal bone loss. (*A*) Bohler angle. (*B*) Crucial angle of Gissane. (*C*) Talar declination angle. (*D*) Talocalcaneal height. (*E*) Talocalcaneal angle.

is performed via a 4-cm incision from the tip of the fibula to the base of the fourth metatarsal. This incision can be used safely, regardless of previous incisions, provided the operation is performed more than 6 months after the index procedure.[46]

In types 2 and 3 malunions, it is necessary to perform a subtalar arthrodesis. As previously mentioned, a standard incision may be used. Frequently, it is possible to perform subtalar arthrodesis with minimal hardware removal (**Fig. 4**). If it is necessary to remove hardware, then it may be performed percutaneously.[47] If bone loss is minimal, then probably an in situ arthrodesis may be performed. However, frequently, although the talar declination angle is normal, CT scan images reveal multiple relatively large cavities around the subtalar joint, which have densely sclerotic walls (**Fig. 5**). It is obviously necessary to debride these cavities back to bleeding cancellous bone. Therefore, although an in situ arthrodesis is being performed, augmentation is necessary to maintain this in situ position. The authors' preference is to use cancellous autograft from the ipsilateral iliac crest, unless there is a contraindication. Orthobiologics (eg, allograft infused with concentrated marrow aspirate) are obviously a viable alternative.

With progressively more-severe bone loss, there are 2 alternative methods of performing the subtalar arthrodesis: in situ and distraction bone block. Larger defects reduce the talocalcaneal height, alter the talocalcaneal angle, and diminish the talar declination angle. In the most severe cases, there is a negative talar declination angle. Carr and colleagues[42] first reported symptomatic ankle impingement secondary to alterations of the talar declination angle in their series of distraction bone block arthrodeses. All cases received a structural bone graft to correct the angular deformity. In this series of 14 patients, the mean talocalcaneal angle improved from 25° to 36° and the mean talar declination angle improved from 14° to 24°. Myerson and Quill[46] described in their large series that the indication for a bone block arthrodesis is a reduction of talocalcaneal height by more than 8 mm. They described good results in 7 patients, fair in 3, and poor in 4. There was a mean increase in ankle dorsiflexion of 15°; it was unchanged in 4 patients and reduced by a mean of 10° in 2 patients. There are several other series that have reported mean postoperative American Orthopaedic

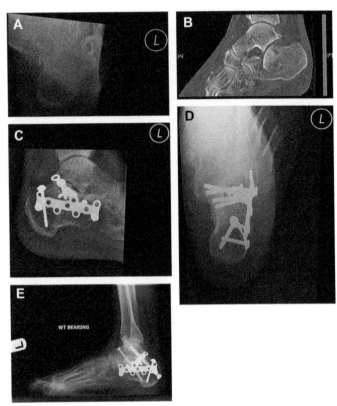

Fig. 4. In situ arthrodesis without hardware removal. (*A*) Pre–open reduction internal fixation (ORIF) axial radiograph. (*B*) Pre-ORIF sagittal CT view. (*C*) Post-ORIF lateral radiograph. (*D*) Post-ORIF axial radiograph. (*E*) Postfusion lateral radiograph.

Foot and Ankle Society (AOFAS) scores of between 64.0 and 76.5.[38,48–53] The change in range of dorsiflexion ranges from an increase of 1° to a decrease of 2°, representing a mean maximum dorsiflexion of 1° to 11°.

Savva and Saxby[40] reported on a series of 17 patients who underwent in situ arthrodesis for subtalar osteoarthritis after calcaneal fracture (type 2 malunion) with marked loss of talocalcaneal height. However, all patients in this series had had the initial fracture treated conservatively. The mean loss of talocalcaneal height was 10.3 mm and the mean talar declination angle was 6.7° (36% of the normal side). The mean postoperative maximum dorsiflexion was 11.6° (almost 80% of the normal side). The mean AOFAS score improved from 29.8 to 77.8. Six patients had heel pain; 6, lateral ankle pain; and 1, anterior ankle pain. No patients had any evidence of anterior ankle impingement. There was a 100% union rate.

Clare and colleagues[36] reported on a series of 45 calcaneal malunions; 30 of these were type 2 malunions and 10 were type 3 malunions. All operations were performed via a lateral extensile approach. Eleven patients (24%) had delayed wound healing, with 1 patient developing a deep infection. Thirty-seven patients (93%) achieved union, with the remaining 3 patients underwent fusion with a revision procedure. The surgical technique was to debride the subtalar joint down to subchondral bone. The joint was then prepared with a 2-mm drill bit. A laminar spreader was then inserted and the jaws opened until the talar head was centered on the navicula. The excised

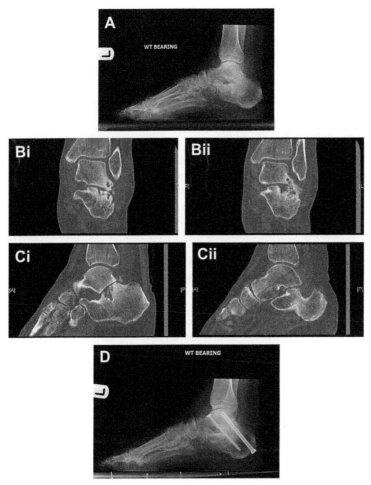

Fig. 5. In situ arthrodesis with large preoperative cavities. (*A*) Preoperative lateral weight-bearing radiograph. (*Bi, Bii*) Preoperative axial CT scan views. (*Ci, Cii*) Preoperative sagittal CT scan views. (*D*) Postfusion lateral weight-bearing radiograph.

lateral wall exostosis was then used as a structural autograft and was augmented with cancellous chips as necessary. The mean postoperative AOFAS score was 74.2; mean talar declination angle, 15.3°; talocalcaneal height, 70.9 mm; and mean dorsiflexion, 12.1°.

In type 3 malunions, Clare and colleagues[36] reported that additional procedures were necessary to correct the deformity within the body of the calcaneus. A Dwyer closing wedge osteotomy was performed for varus malalignment and a medial displacement osteotomy for valgus deformities. Results in type 3 malunions were reported as a mean AOFAS score of 76.1, mean dorsiflexion of 7.5°, mean talar declination angle of 7.5%, and talocalcaneal height of 76.2 mm.

The authors' preferred technique for subtalar arthrodesis in both types 2 and 3 malunions is in situ arthrodesis. These malunions are augmented with cancellous autograft, unless very little is sclerosis present preoperatively. A 6.5-mm long partially threaded titanium screw is placed from the non–weight-bearing surface of the posterior calcaneus into the talus, with the entry point being just proximal to the start of the skin of the plantar surface of the foot. A second wire is then driven parallel but 2 cm anteriorly through the calcaneus and talus and out through the skin (avoiding the neurovascular bundle). A 4-mm partially threaded titanium cancellous screw is then passed in a retrograde manner (**Fig. 6**). However, if ankle impingement was evident on the preoperative lateral weight-bearing forced dorsiflexion and plantar-flexion radiographs, distraction arthrodesis is performed using the methods described in the next section.

Treatment of nonunions

Nonunion is a rarely reported complication of calcaneal fractures. There are 5 reports totaling 7 patients in the literature; only 1 had a nonunion of the body of the calcaneus, which was successfully treated with open reduction internal fixation.[54–58] Molloy and colleagues[45] reported on a series of 15 nonunions. About 93% of these nonunions had been initially treated in other institutions with open reduction internal fixation. However, in 86% of patients the initial reduction and placement of hardware was poor. Three cases (20%) were complicated by chronic osteomyelitis and 3 (20%) by wound dehiscence without infection. The mean preoperative Bohler angle was 9.3°, and the mean talar declination angle was 8.3° (−20° to 2.5°). All patients had subtalar arthritis, and 20% had concomitant calcaneocuboid arthritis. All patients received allograft. In situ arthrodeses were performed through an incision from the tip of the fibula to the base of the fourth metatarsal, and distraction bone block arthrodeses were approached via a retrofibular incision (67%). Of the 12 noninfected cases, 6 (50%) healed after the first procedure, with the remaining 50% undergoing fusion after

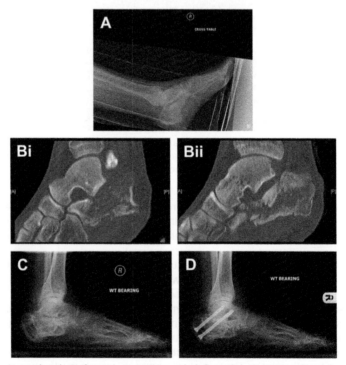

Fig. 6. In situ arthrodesis for a large calcaneal defect. (*A*) Postinjury lateral radiograph. (*Bi, Bii*) Postinjury sagittal CT views. (*C*) Prearthrodesis lateral weight-bearing radiograph. (*D*) Postfusion lateral weight-bearing radiograph.

revisional procedures. Two patients needed abductor flaps for wound dehiscence, but both these patients previously also had wound dehiscences after their primary procedure. The 3 infected cases had the infection successfully eradicated by staged procedures. Two cases underwent fusion successfully. In 1 patient, symptoms were sufficiently controlled with cement spacer in situ after the primary procedure (AOFAS score, 88), so the patient declined further treatment. The eventual outcome was a subtalar fusion in 10 patients and a triple arthrodesis in 4 patients. The mean AOFAS score was 69 (range, 40–88), and the mean talar declination angle was 21°.

If possible, a subtalar arthrodesis alone is performed. However, if there is symptomatic calcaneocuboid arthritis, triple arthrodesis should be performed. This procedure should also be followed if the distal fragment of the calcaneal neck is less than 2 cm in length anteroposteriorly because reliable and reproducible stability of internal fixation is extremely challenging if internal fixation rather than arthrodesis was to be performed. For triple arthrodesis, the calcaneocuboid and talonavicular arthrodeses are performed in a standard fashion; however, if there is a distal nonunion of the calcaneus, the calcaneocuboid arthrodesis fixation may be supplemented with a spanning locking plate.

The authors' preference is to carry out an in situ arthrodesis and revision of the nonunion. This approach is normally via a standard lateral approach from the tip of the fibula to the base of the fourth metatarsal. It is, however, imperative that there is sufficiently accurate preoperative imaging, so that assessment of the size of the potential defect caused by nonviable bone can be made. If there is painful anterior ankle impingement or severe bone loss, then a distraction bone block arthrodesis is performed via a retrofibular incision. This is because distraction produces tension in a longitudinal plane, which would contribute to wound healing problems if a standard lateral incision or extensile lateral approach is used. If a triple arthrodesis is to be performed, then a separate lateral longitudinal incision may be used because it will be outside the plane of tension.

Whichever approach is used, the metalwork is first removed, and then the nonunion is addressed. There is usually partial (or at least fibrous) union present. Thorough debridement of all fibrous tissue and avascular bone is undertaken. The aim is that there should be at least punctate bleeding at the debridement margins, which is not sometimes possible distally where dense sclerosis may be present. Preparation is then performed with a 2-mm drill bit. Augmentation is always used in this scenario, and autograft/allograft together with concentrated marrow aspirate should be used.

The subtalar joint is next addressed by the same methods of thorough debridement. If an in situ arthrodesis is to be performed, then some cancellous autograft is still used. Fixation is achieved for the arthrodesis and across the nonunion using 6.5- or 8-mm partially threaded titanium cannulated screws. A low-profile locking plate can be added for further stability. If there is gross comminution of the nonunion, multiple smaller diameter screws may be necessary. For a distraction arthrodesis, a laminar spreader is inserted into the defect. The jaws are opened by pressing against both the subtalar joint side of the talus and the calcaneal tuberosity. This distraction corrects the medial column alignment toward normality (**Fig. 7**). If the defect is very large, then Achilles tendon lengthening may be necessary to be able to relatively depress the calcaneal tuberosity. The authors' preference in a distraction arthrodesis is to only perform enough distraction so as to prevent ankle impingement and to achieve acceptable hindfoot and midfoot alignment rather than to achieve absolute anatomic normality so as to reduce the chance of wound problems (delayed healing, dehiscence, and infection). The defect must then be filled with graft; either a tricortical iliac autograft with cancellous autograft packed around it or an allograft infused with platelet-rich plasma/concentrated bone marrow aspirate.

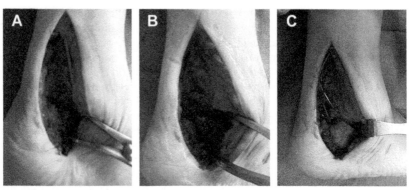

Fig. 7. Distraction bone block arthrodesis. (*A*) After debridement. (*B*) Distraction of the defect with laminar spreader. (*C*) Insertion of allograft.

OPEN INJURIES

Severe crush injuries and blast injuries may produce extremely challenging open injuries in the calcaneus. The latter are associated with more extensive soft tissue injuries as well as concomitant peripheral and core injuries. The most important part of the decision-making process is whether to perform a primary amputation or limb salvage. Indications for amputation are transaction of the tibial nerve and irreparable vascular injury.[59] The treatment of open calcaneal fractures follows the same principles as any other significant open injury. Thorough debridement of devitalized tissue and avascular bone (no matter how extensive the fragment is) is mandatory. Obviously thorough debridement and lavage of any contaminating material from the wound (which is normally plantar medial) is necessary. Initial stabilization also needs to be achieved. In the civilian setting, this process usually involves a bridging external fixator. Application of negative pressure dressings is extremely useful for producing an aseptic seal and promoting granulation tissue. They can provide valuable time for planning definitive fixation and wound coverage, in conjunction with plastic surgical colleagues.

The overall treatment of massive calcaneal bone loss from blast injuries in the military setting is highly specialized. The most appropriate opinion on this treatment is from the laudable military staff who carry out such treatments in active service. Therefore, readers are referred to the articles by Shawen and colleagues[59] and Keeling and colleagues.[60]

SUMMARY

Massive bone loss following calcaneal fractures is a challenging condition to treat, especially if nonunion is present. Meticulous preoperative examination and imaging are crucial for accurate preoperative planning. If performed, successful outcomes can be achieved with the strategies outlined in this article.

REFERENCES

1. McBride DJ, Ramamurthy C, Laing P. The hindfoot: calcaneal and talar fractures and dislocations-Part I fractures of the calcaneum. Curr Orthop 2005;19:94–100.
2. Allmacher D, Galles K, Marsh J. Intra-articular calcaneal fractures treated nonoperatively and followed sequentially for 2 decades. J Orthop Trauma 2006;20(7): 464–9.

3. Ibrahim T, Rowsell M, Rennie M, et al. Displaced intra-articular calcaneal fractures: 15-year follow-up of a randomised controlled trial of conservative versus operative treatment. Injury 2007;38(7):848–55.
4. Parmar H, Triffit P, Gregg P. Intra-articular fractures of the calcaneum treated operatively or conservatively. J Bone Joint Surg Br 1993;75:932–7.
5. Randle J, Kreder H, Stephen D, et al. Should calcaneal fractures be treated surgically? A meta-analysis. Clin Orthop 2000;377:217–27.
6. Bajammal S, Tornetta P, Sanders D, et al. Displaced intra-articular calcaneal fractures. J Orthop Trauma 2005;19(5):360–4.
7. Rammelt S, Gavlik J, Barthel S, et al. The value of subtalar arthroscopy in the management of intra-articular calcaneus fractures. Foot Ankle Int 2002;23(10):906–15.
8. Eastwood D, Gregg P, Atkins R. Intra-articular fractures of the calcaneum. J Bone Joint Surg Br 1993;75:183–8.
9. Eastwood D, Langkamer V, Atkins R. Intra-articular fractures of the calcaneum. J Bone Joint Surg Br 1993;75:189–95.
10. Schepers T, Vogels L, Schipper I, et al. Percutaneous reduction and fixation of intraarticular calcaneal fractures. Oper Orthop Traumatol 2008;20:168–75.
11. Zwipp H, Tscherne H, Thermann H, et al. Osteosynthesis of displaced intraarticular fractures of the calcaneus. Clin Orthop Relat Res 1993;290:76–86.
12. Bridgman S, Dunn K, McBride D, et al. Interventions for treating calcaneal fractures. Cochrane Database Syst Rev 2000;2:CD001161.
13. Leung K, Yeun K, Chan K. Operative treatment of displaced intra-articular fractures of the calcaneum. J Bone Joint Surg Br 1993;75:196–201.
14. Loucks C, Buckley R. Bohler's angle: correlation with outcome in displaced intra-articular calcaneal fractures. J Orthop Trauma 1999;13(8):554–8.
15. Crosby L, Fitzgibbons T. Intraarticular calcaneal fractures. Results of closed treatment. Clin Orthop Relat Res 1993;290:47–54.
16. Paul M, Peter R, Hoffmeyer P. Fractures of the calcaneum. J Bone Joint Surg Br 2004;86:1142–5.
17. Barla J, Buckley R, McCormack R, et al. Displaced intraarticular calcaneal fractures: long-term outcome in women. Foot Ankle Int 2004;25(12):853–6.
18. Tennent T, Calder P, Salisbury R, et al. The operative management of displaced intra-articular fractures of the calcaneum: a two-centre study using a defined protocol. Injury 2001;32:491–6.
19. Hutchinson F, Huebner M. Treatment of os calcis fractures by open reduction internal fixation. Foot Ankle Int 1994;15(5):225–32.
20. Csizy M, Buckley R, Tough S, et al. Displaced intra-articular calcaneal fractures: variables predicting late subtalar fusion. J Orthop Trauma 2003;17(2):106–12.
21. Herscovici D, Widmaier J, Scaduto J, et al. Operative treatment of calcaneal fractures in elderly patients. J Bone Joint Surg Am 2005;87(6):1260–4.
22. Basile A. Operative versus nonoperative treatment of displaced intra-articular calcaneal fractures in elderly patients. J Foot Ankle Surg 2010;49(1):25–32.
23. Howard J, Buckley R, McCormack R, et al. Complications following management of displaced intra-articular calcaneal fractures: a prospective randomized trial comparing open reduction internal fixation with nonoperative management. J Orthop Trauma 2003;17(4):241–9.
24. Buckley R, Tough S, McCormack R, et al. Operative compared with non-operative management of displaced intra-articular calcaneal fractures. J Bone Joint Surg Br 2002;84(10):1733–43.

25. O'Brien J, Buckley R, McCormack R, et al. Personal gait satisfaction after displaced intraarticular calcaneal fractures: a 2–8 year followup. Foot Ankle Int 2004;25(9):657–73.
26. Catani F, Benedetti M, Simoncini L, et al. Analysis of function after intra-articular fracture of the os calcis. Foot Ankle Int 1999;20(7):417–21.
27. Kingwell S, Buckley R, Willis N. The association between subtalar joint motion and outcome satisfaction in patients with displaced intraarticular calcaneal fractures. Foot Ankle Int 2004;25(9):666–73.
28. Talarico L, Vito G, Zyryanov S. Management of displaced intraarticular calcaneal fractures by using external ring fixation, minimally invasive open reduction, and early weightbearing. J Foot Ankle Surg 2004;43(1):43–50.
29. McGarvey W, Burris M, Clanton T, et al. Calcaneal fractures: indirect reduction and external fixation. Foot Ankle Int 2006;27(7):494–9.
30. Emara K, Allam F. Management of calcaneal fracture using the Ilizarov technique. Clin Orthop Relat Res 2005;439:215–20.
31. Rammelt S, Amlang M, Barthel S, et al. Minimally invasive treatment of calcaneal fractures. Injury 2004;35(Suppl 2):SB55–63.
32. Tufescu T, Buckley R. Age, gender, work capability, and worker's compensation in patients with displaced intraarticular calcaneal fractures. J Orthop Trauma 2001; 15(4):275–9.
33. O'Farrell D, O'Byrne J, McCabe J, et al. Fractures of the os calcis: improved results with internal fixation. Injury 1993;24(4):263–5.
34. Kundel K, Funk E, Brutscher M, et al. Calcaneal fractures: operative versus nonoperative treatment. J Trauma 1996;41(5):839–45.
35. Robinson J, Murphy A. Arthrodesis as salvage for calcaneal malunions. Foot Ankle Clin 2002;7:107–20.
36. Clare M, Lee W, Sanders R. Intermediate to long-term results of a treatment protocol for calcaneal fracture malunions. J Bone Joint Surg Am 2005;87:963–73.
37. Reddy V, Fukuda T, Ptaszek A. Calcaneus malunion and non-union. Foot Ankle Clin 2007;12:125–35.
38. Flemister A, Infante A, Sanders R, et al. Subtalar arthrodesis for complications of intra-articular calcaneal fractures. Foot Ankle Int 2000;21(5):392–9.
39. Huang P-J, Fu Y-C, Cheng Y-M, et al. Subtalar arthrodesis for late sequelae of calcaneal fractures: fusion in situ versus fusion with sliding corrective osteotomy. Foot Ankle Int 1999;20(3):166–70.
40. Savva N, Saxby T. In situ arthrodesis with lateral-wall ostectomy for sequelae of fracture of the os calcis. J Bone Joint Surg Br 2007;89(7):919–24.
41. Stephens HM, Sanders R. Calcaneal malunions: results of a prognostic computed tomography classification system. Foot Ankle Int 1996;17:395–401.
42. Carr JV, Hansen ST, Benirschke SK. Subtalar distraction bone block arthrodesis for complications of os calcis fractures. Foot Ankle 1988;9:81–6.
43. Gallie WE. Subastralger arthrodesis in fractures of the os calcis. J Bone Joint Surg Br 1943;25(4):731–6.
44. Barei DP, Bellasbarba C, Sangeorzan BJ, et al. Fractures of the calcaneus. Orthop Clin North Am 2002;33:263–85.
45. Molloy AP, Myerson MS, Yoon P. Symptomatic non-union after fracture of the calcaneum. Demographics and treatment. J Bone Joint Surg Br 2007;89:1218–24.
46. Myerson M, Quill GE Jr. Late complication of fractures of the calcaneus. J Bone Joint Surg Am 1993;75:331–41.
47. Stamatis ED, Myerson MS. Percutaneous hardware removal after open reduction and internal fixation of calcaneus fractures. Orthopedics 2002;25:1025–7.

48. Bednarz PA, Beals TC, Manoli A 2nd. Subtalar distraction bone block fusion: an assessment of outcome. Foot Ankle Int 1997;18:785–91.
49. Burton DC, Olney BW, Horton GA. Late results of subtalar distraction fusion. Foot Ankle Int 1998;19:197–202.
50. Easley ME, Trnka HJ, Schon LC, et al. Isolated subtalar arthrodesis. J Bone Joint Surg Am 2000;82:613–24.
51. Chan SC, Alexander IJ. Subtalar arthrodesis with interposition tricortical iliac crest bone graft for late pain and deformity after calcaneus fracture. Foot Ankle Int 1997;18:613–5.
52. Rammelt S, Grass R, Zawadski T, et al. Foot function after distraction bone-block arthrodesis. J Bone Joint Surg Br 2004;86:659–68.
53. Trnka HJ, Easley ME, Lam PW, et al. Subtalar distraction bone block arthrodesis. J Bone Joint Surg Br 2001;83:849–54.
54. Robbins MI, Wilson MG, Sella EJ. MR imaging of anterosuperior calcaneal process fractures. AJR AM J Roentgenol 1999;172:475–9.
55. Levine J, Kenin A, Spinner M. Non-union of a fracture of the anterior superior process of the calcaneus. J Bone Joint Surg Am 1959;41:178–80.
56. Piatt AB. Fractures of the promontory of the calcaneus. Radiology 1956;67:386–91.
57. Myerson MS, Berger BI. Non-union of a fracture of the sustentaculum tali causin tarsal tunnel syndrome: a case report. Foot Ankle Int 1995;16:740–2.
58. Thomas P, Wilson LF. Non-union of an os calcis fracture. Injury 1993;24:630–2.
59. Shawen SB, Keeling JJ, Branstetter J, et al. The mangled foot and leg: salvage versus amputation. Foot Ankle Clin 2010;15:63–75.
60. Keeling JJ, Hsu JR, Shawen SB, et al. Strategies for managing massive defects of the foot in high-energy combat injuries of the lower extremity. Foot Ankle Clin 2010;15:139–49.

A Novel Surgical Technique for the Management of Massive Osseous Defects in the Hindfoot with Bulk Allograft

Brian E. Clowers, MD, Mark S. Myerson, MD*

KEYWORDS

• Arthrodesis • Hindfoot • Femoral head • Allograft

Tibiotalocalcaneal (TTC) arthrodesis is a procedure that allows for the simultaneous treatment of end-stage ankle and hindfoot arthritides. The procedure offers a surgeon the ability to simultaneously manage hindfoot and ankle pathology while sparing the transverse tarsal joint, which is an advantage over a pantalar fusion.[1] Furthermore, this procedure provides the surgeon the ability to correct significant hindfoot and ankle malalignment. In many cases, concomitant hindfoot and ankle arthritides arise secondary to frank collapse of the talar body, such as is seen with Charcot arthropathy in the diabetic or neuropathic patient, or in the setting of avascular necrosis of the talus, commonly encountered in the posttraumatic setting.[2,3] However, the procedure is not always straightforward because of the effects these pathologies have on the bony structure of the talus.[1,4,5]

In a setting that necessitates a fusion of both the ankle joint and the hindfoot, it is common to encounter a massive osseous defect, specifically of the talus, such as is created by the previously discussed pathologies. Large bony defects present a problem because simple excision of the collapsed bone and fusion of the remaining structures result in significant shortening of the limb. It is desirable to maintain the length of the hindfoot, both to preserve the overall length of the limb and to avoid soft tissue complications, and this requires the use of a structural allograft to fill the void left by the vacated talar body. Routinely, a structural allograft for the hindfoot consists of a piece of femoral head allograft cut into a block shape that is used to

The Institute for Foot and Ankle Reconstruction, Mercy Medical Center, Baltimore, 301 St Paul Place, Baltimore, MD 21202, USA
* Corresponding author.
E-mail address: mark4feet@aol.com

recreate the talar body. We present an alternative and a novel surgical technique that uses the entire femoral head allograft as the block graft, in addition to a unique manner of preparation of the tibial and/or calcaneal articular surfaces.

SURGICAL TECHNIQUE
Graft Preparation

Traditionally, when a massive osseous defect dictates the use of a bulk cortical allograft (**Fig. 1**A), a block is cut from a femoral head allograft to approximate the shape of the residual bony defect. Commonly, the block is cut into the shape of a trapezoid consisting of flat surfaces, which provides broad cancellous surfaces with adequate surface area to optimize healing and stability at the native bone–allograft interface (see **Fig. 1**B). In addition, this block allows for maintenance of the length of the limb by filling the defect left by the body of the talus.

Instead of a cut block portion of the femoral head/neck, we propose the use of the entire spherical portion of the femoral head allograft in conjunction with a unique joint preparation technique that is discussed later. To prepare the graft, the neck portion of the allograft is resected with a sagittal saw, leaving a spherical graft (**Fig. 2**). A sagittal saw or rasp is then used to contour the cut surface of the graft to make it as rounded as possible, while also paring the size of the graft to fit the size of the osseous defect. The femoral head allograft comes with the articular surface denuded of its cartilage, leaving a graft with a circumferentially cancellous surface once the femoral neck and calcar are resected. A 2-mm drill is then used to perforate the entire surface of the spherical allograft (**Fig. 3**).[1] Iliac crest stem cell aspirate is then injected into the inner cancellous substance of the spherical graft, and the outer surface of the graft is coated in the iliac crest stem cell aspirate (**Fig. 4**).[1]

Joint Preparation

With the use of a spherical allograft, a new joint preparation technique must also be used to accomplish the 2 main goals of the preparation: (1) creating a mated articular

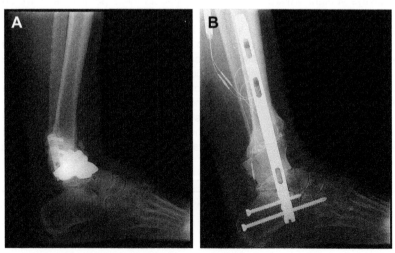

Fig. 1. (*A*) This patient had a failed total ankle with avascular necrosis and collapse of the talus, (*B*) which was managed with a standard trapezoidal structural allograft and a hindfoot nail.

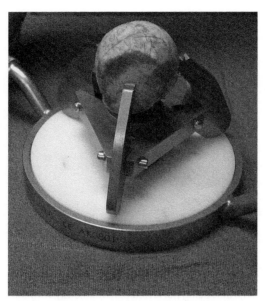

Fig. 2. A bulk femoral head allograft with the neck and calcar portion resected, leaving a spherical graft. The cartilage has been denuded, and cancellous surfaces are exposed.

surface that fits the shape of the spherical graft and (2) debriding the native articular surfaces of cartilage and sclerotic bone so that a fresh cancellous surface is exposed to the allograft.[2] We accomplish both of these goals with the use of an acetabular reamer. Joint preparation with a reamer can be performed through a standard

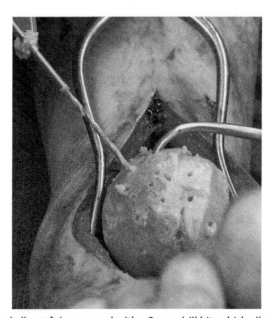

Fig. 3. The spherical allograft is prepared with a 2-mm drill bit, which allows for penetration of osteogenic adjuvants, such as iliac crest aspirate.

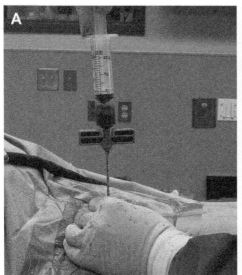
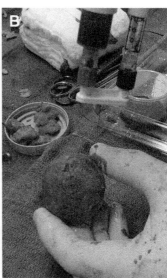

Fig. 4. (*A*) Iliac crest adjuvant being harvested percutaneously with the use of a cannulated trocar. (*B*) Aspirate as applied to the spherical graft, coating the outer surface of the graft and penetrating into the prepared drill holes.

transfibular approach or also by way of an anterior approach, based on the surgeon's preference, previous surgical procedures/incisions, and the deformity that is present. Reaming of the distal tibia and the posterior facet of the calcaneus takes the place of the more standard technique of flat saw cuts across the distal tibia and the calcaneal facet, which generally accompanies the use of a trapezoidal block allograft.

The acetabular reaming instrumentation consists of a hemispheric reamer that can be attached to a drive shaft and a power drive (**Fig. 5**). We generally use a 36-mm diameter reamer, one of the smaller-diameter reamers available, allowing the surgeon a great deal of freedom and the ability to contour the shape of the distal tibia and posterior facet

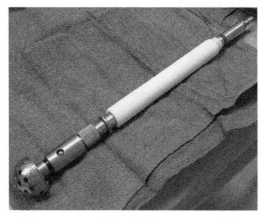

Fig. 5. A 36-mm acetabular reamer and drive shaft apparatus, which is attached to a power driver when ready for use.

based on the patient's anatomic features. Once again, the goal of the joint preparation is to create a concave surface that accommodates the femoral head allograft and its convex contour and to create a cancellous surface that promotes bony healing between the native bone and the allograft. The reaming technique offers the surgeon flexibility and forgiveness because it is not necessary to exactly match the radius of curvature of the femoral head allograft to the reamed concavity and make the precise bone cuts that are required by the standard bone block technique.[5] The combination of the reaming technique and the spherical graft also gives the surgeon the ability to correct sagittal, coronal, and axial plane deformities very quickly and easily. Spherical interfaces allow the surgeon to "dial in" the alignment and position of the foot without needing to revise the preparation of the joint surfaces.

With the first pass of the reamer, the joint surfaces are denuded of cartilage and scar tissue as well as the subchondral bone, which is often sclerotic. Specifically, the reamer is run in the forward direction (eg, clockwise) and is started before applying it to the bony surface (**Fig. 6**). Starting the reamer before contact with the bone is crucial to prevent binding of the reamer and to prevent damage to the native cortical and cancellous surfaces. With the reamer running, it is gently applied to the distal tibia or calcaneus, and then moderate pressure is applied axially to the reamer/driver apparatus. Once the cartilage and sclerotic bone are denuded, the reamer is cleaned and emptied of debris and then applied again to the cancellous bony surfaces in similar fashion, where it can be used to prepare the distal tibia and the posterior facet of the calcaneus by sculpting the cancellous bone into a smooth concave surface (**Fig. 7**). Care must be taken at this point not to apply too much pressure to the reamer because the reaming blades are sharp and an excessive amount of bone can be removed very easily. At this time, morselized cancellous autograft can also be removed from the basket of the reamer and saved for later use at the allograft/native bone interfaces (**Fig. 8**).[2]

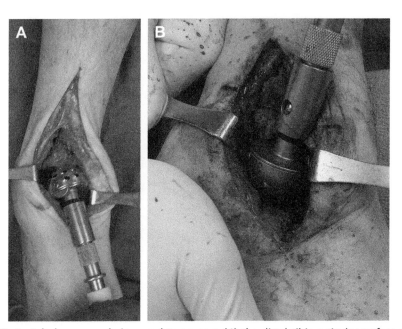

Fig. 6. Acetabular reamer being used to prepare (A) the distal tibia articular surface and (B) the posterior facet of the calcaneus.

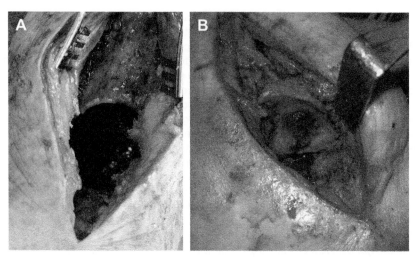

Fig. 7. (*A, B*) Joint surfaces after being prepared with the reamer. Note the smooth contour of the prepared surface, which generally mirrors the shape of the spherical graft and the exposed bleeding cancellous bone.

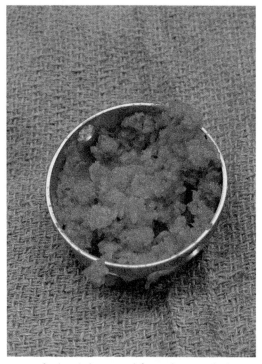

Fig. 8. Morselized autograft that is harvested from the acetabular reamer. The autograft can be applied to the allograft–native bone interface to augment the allograft.

The joint surfaces are adequately prepared once healthy bleeding cancellous bone is visible and when the shape of the prepared joint surface accommodates the shape of the femoral head spherical allograft. The allograft should fit easily but securely into the prepared cavity and should be able to be positioned correctly without the need for excessive force (**Fig. 9**). Conversely, there should not be significant space between the graft and the prepared joint surfaces. Autograft obtained from the reaming of the joint surfaces can be packed into any spaces left remaining between the native cancellous bone and the allograft. With the graft in place, the hindfoot and ankle can be positioned properly in the sagittal, coronal, and axial planes in preparation for provisional and definitive fixations. The position of the graft and alignment of the ankle and hindfoot should be confirmed with multiplanar fluoroscopy before fixation (**Fig. 10**).

Fixation

Our technique does not demand any different type of fixation when compared with the standard TTC or talocalcaneal fusion, and we still recommend the use of an intramedullary nail (**Fig. 11**)[3] or a blade plate implant.[2] Cannulated screws remain an option, but the aforementioned implants are technically simpler and provide more inherent stability than screws alone because they both can function as fixed-angle devices. An intramedullary device also offers the advantage of serving as a load-sharing device, which has a theoretic advantage over a load-bearing device when bony healing is desired in a weight-bearing location.

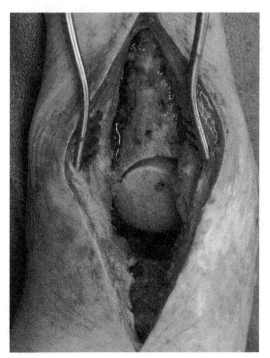

Fig. 9. The spherical graft in place after preparation of the native joint surfaces. Note that the graft fits easily into the prepared space and can be positioned without difficulty.

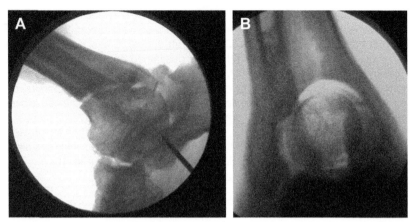

Fig. 10. (*A, B*) Fluoroscopic image of the spherical graft in place to confirm the alignment of the hindfoot and the position of the graft.

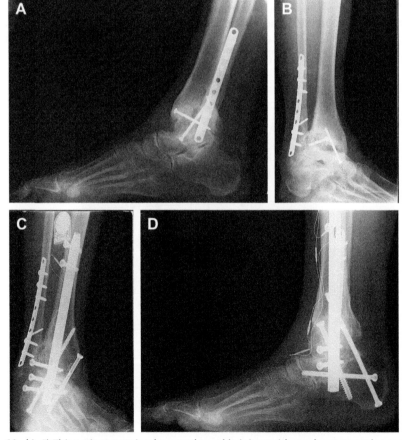

Fig. 11. (*A, B*) This patient sustained a complex ankle injury with resultant avascular necrosis of the talus. (*C, D*) A talocalcaneal arthrodesis with a hindfoot nail and a spherical allograft was performed in the patient.

SUMMARY

The use of a spherical femoral head allograft in conjunction with spherical reaming provides a safe and effective technique for the management of a massive osseous defect in the hindfoot. This technique presents specific advantages over the standard technique of trapezoidal block allograft and joint preparation by way of flat osteotomies, including increased flexibility and freedom in deformity correction and joint alignment. The technique can be used in concert with standard surgical approaches and fixation techniques and uses instrumentation that is readily available. To this point, we have experienced comparable surgical outcomes with this technique when compared with the standard approach.

REFERENCES

1. Myerson MS. Tibiotalocalcaneal and pan-talar arthrodesis. In: Myerson MS, editor. Reconstructive foot and ankle surgery: management of complications. 2nd edition. Philadelphia: Elsevier Saunders; 2010. p. 505–17.
2. Myerson MS, Alvarez RG, Lam PW. Tibiocalcaneal arthrodesis for the management of severe ankle and hindfoot deformities. Foot Ankle Int 2000;21:643–50.
3. Niinimaki TT, Klemola TM, Leppilahti JI. Tibiotalocalcaneal arthrodesis with a compressive retrograde intramedullary nail: a report of 34 consecutive patients. Foot Ankle Int 2007;28:431–4.
4. Papa JA, Myerson MS. Pantalar and tibiotalocalcaneal arthrodesis for post-traumatic osteoarthrosis of the ankle and hindfoot. J Bone Joint Surg Am 1992; 74:1042–9.
5. Papa J, Myerson MS, Girard P. Salvage, with arthrodesis, in intractable diabetic neuropathic arthropathy of the foot and ankle. J Bone Joint Surg Am 1993;75: 1056–66.

Index

Note: Page numbers of article titles are in **boldface** type.

Foot Ankle Clin N Am 16 (2011) 191–211

doi:10.1016/S1083-7515(11)00014-3

1083-7515/11/$ – see front matter © 2011 Elsevier Inc. All rights reserved.

foot.theclinics.com

Moving?

Make sure your subscription moves with you!

To notify us of your new address, find your **Clinics Account Number** (located on your mailing label above your name), and contact customer service at:

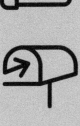

Email: journalscustomerservice-usa@elsevier.com

800-654-2452 (subscribers in the U.S. & Canada)
314-447-8871 (subscribers outside of the U.S. & Canada)

Fax number: 314-447-8029

Elsevier Health Sciences Division
Subscription Customer Service
3251 Riverport Lane
Maryland Heights, MO 63043

*To ensure uninterrupted delivery of your subscription, please notify us at least 4 weeks in advance of move.

Printed and bound by CPI Group (UK) Ltd, Croydon, CR0 4YY

03/10/2024

01040460-0003